KATHARINA BRINKMANN

Fascial Fitness through Yoga

WITH
A COMPREHENSIVE
CATALOGUE OF EXERCISES
AND THE
FASCIA SALUTATION

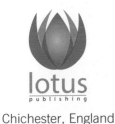

lotus
publishing

Chichester, England

First published by Riva Verlag, rivaverlag,de. All rights reserved. This English language edition published in 2018 by Lotus Publishing, Apple Tree Cottage, Inlands Road, Nutbourne, Chichester, PO18 8RJ.

Picture credits: Shutterstock: P. 5, 11, 12, 13, 17, 31, 33–43, 45–46, 127
Photos: squaredotmedia GbR, www.squaredot.media

Editing: Frauke Bahle
Cover design: Isabella Dorsch
Cover illustrations: squaredotmedia GbR
Layout and typesetting: Katja Muggli, www.katjamuggli.de
Printing: Everbest Printing Co. Ltd.
Printed in China

ISBN 978 1 905367 83 2

You can find more information on the publisher at lotuspublishing.co.uk

Contents

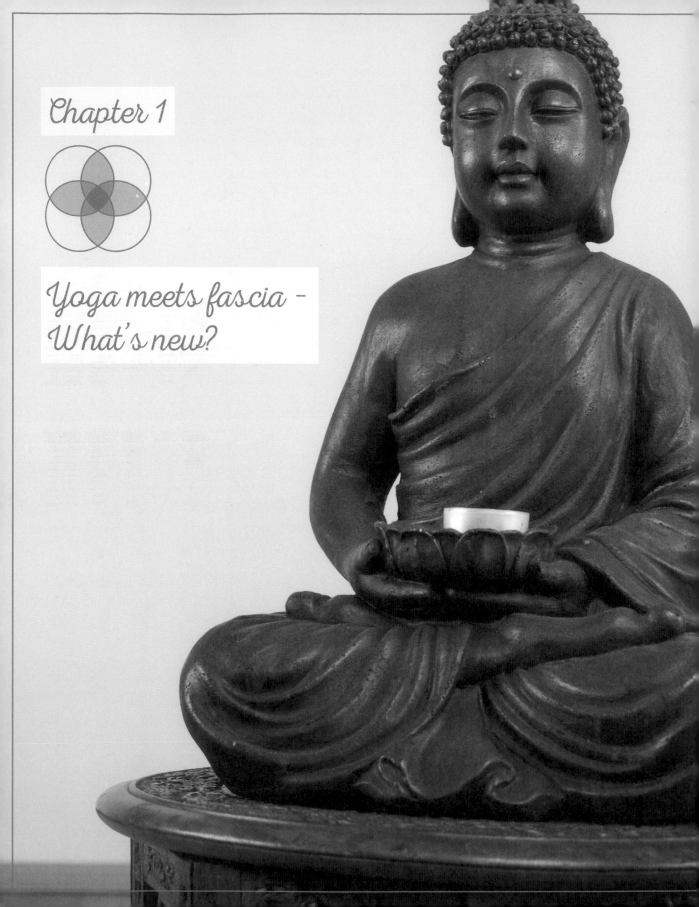

Chapter 1

Yoga meets fascia - What's new?

At first glance, fascia training and yoga philosophy seem to be two completely different things. Fascia research – a modern field of research, still in its infancy – aims to shed light on the manifestations and functions of fascia, and establish anatomical and physiological connections. Yoga is an ancient Indian teaching on movement and living that incorporates the holistic energetic body and spirit. Yoga is based on thousands of years of teaching and experience, which evolved from the experience and perception of movement. Two approaches that couldn't be more different. But, as you will see, the worlds of yoga and fascia share common ground. What yogis have experienced for thousands of years can now be made tangible and explained through science.

Why fascia yoga?

Yoga is fascia training! Even traditional yoga poses provide excellent fascia training, as they stretch long muscle chains. Fascia likes to be pulled and stretched, as is the case in yoga. And it is a real motion artist, requiring a variety of movements – both flexible bouncing movements and slower, almost imperceptible pulsing. Fascia is probably the most diverse tissue in our bodies, and the ways of training it are just as diverse. In fascia yoga, fascial tissue is taken much further than simple stretching. Fascia yoga focuses your yoga practice on fascial tissues, making your body more supple and offering a creative new approach to traditional yoga. In contrast to traditional, static yoga styles, in fascia yoga you are rarely in one position for longer than a few breaths.

Creativity and openness to new movement patterns, an enjoyment of the act of moving and a focus on external and internal "chains" characterise this "fascia-nating" style of yoga!

What is fascia yoga?

Fascia yoga is a style of yoga that is rich in movement and variety, focusing on probably the most interesting tissues in our body. It is composed of several building blocks that reach the fascial network on all levels. Think of these building blocks as the petals of a magnificent flower. Each petal has its own raison d'être and its own individual charm. Each petal makes the flower complete, and together they form a unit – fascia yoga.

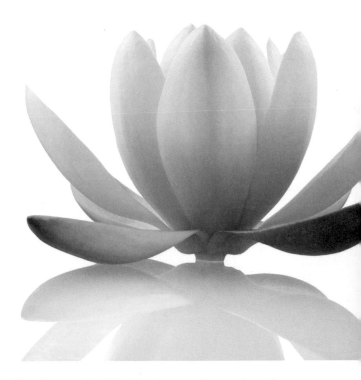

The five petals of the fascia yoga flower stand for the five training elements we find in fascia yoga. In chapters 4 to 8, you will find more information on how to implement this practice and its scientific background. But for now, here's a quick overview of what you can expect:

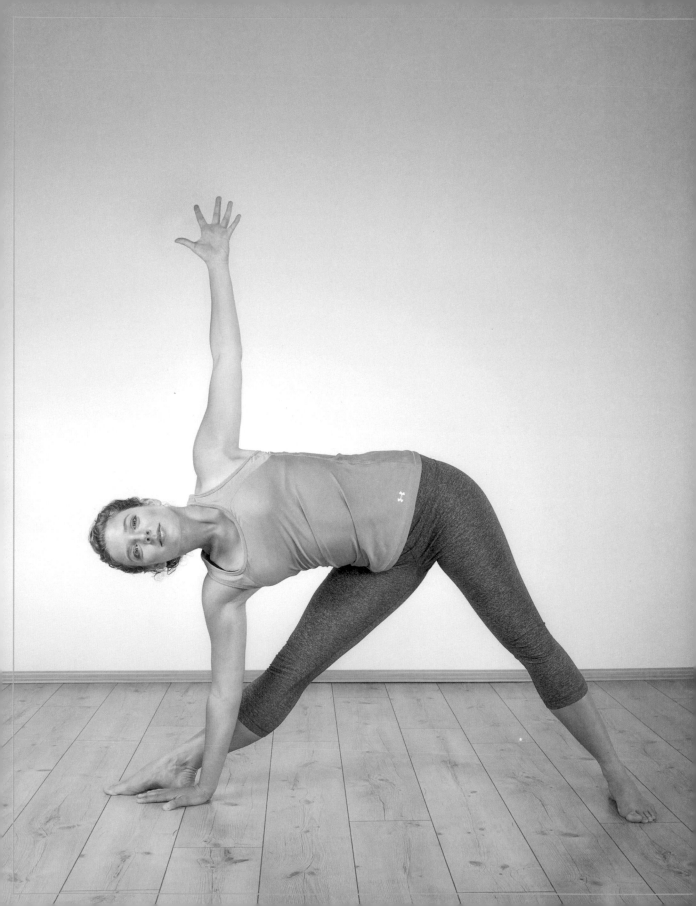

Tension release *(chapter 4)*
Indulge yourself with a mini self-massage to prepare for your yoga practice, or to recuperate after an intensive session. With the fascia roller and ball, you can smooth out your fascial tissues and loosen "stuck" areas.

Fascial stretching *(chapter 5)*
Fascia likes to be stretched – particularly in all directions and over the longest possible myofascial chains. In this chapter, you will learn how to make traditional yoga poses even more "fascia-friendly".

Strong and stable *(chapter 6)*
Centring plays an important role in yoga, particularly in standing and balancing poses. In this chapter, we focus on the deep frontal fascial chain, as this provides stability and body tension.

Elasticity *(chapter 7)*
The ability to conserve energy, like a catapult or a spring, is one of the most interesting properties of fascia. In this chapter, you will spring, rock, swing, bounce and jump. Discover the possibilities the world of yoga has to offer.

Breathing *(chapter 8)*
In terms of physiology, breathing is also a form of fascia training. But how often are you really breathing with awareness? In this chapter, explore the theory and practice of how you can reach the fascia just by breathing in your yoga practice and your daily life.

What can fascia yoga do for you?

Fascia yoga brings the fascial network into balance. It takes a holistic approach, uniting the physical body with the mind and the soul.

Fascia yoga

» keeps your fascial network supple and elastic, and at the same time provides stability and resistance.
» promotes awareness of the body and nurtures the senses. You will get in touch with your self and discover new ranges of motion.
» invites you to be curious and creative.
» can help with pain, tension and injury. There are many receptors of all kinds in fascia, particularly in the back.
» is fun!

Please note, fascia yoga is not a universal remedy. But it is a wonderful opportunity to get to know your own body better.

 The word "yoga" comes from the root "yuj", which essentially means "to join" or "to unite". The merging of body, mind and soul is the overarching concept in yoga. This unity is also reflected in our fascial network, as our fascia is also interconnected.

What is yoga?

Yoga is a comprehensive concept that covers much more than a physical method of relaxation. It is deeply rooted in Indian culture and tradition, and can be considered as a holistic system that brings the body, mind and soul into harmony. It is generally accepted that the classical yoga tradition began with the Yoga Sutras of Patanjali. Around 2000 years ago, Patanjali described the eight components of yoga with practical techniques and methods for achieving the goal of yoga – knowledge of the self. This view is still relevant today, and is incorporated into the practice of fascia yoga.

Patanjali's eightfold yoga path

» Yama: dealing with the world

» Niyama: dealing with the self

» Asanas: physical exercises

» Pranayama: regulation of the breathing

» Pratyahara: withdrawal of the senses

» Dharana: concentration

» Dhyana: meditation

» Samadhi: enlightenment

Over time, many different types and traditions of yoga have developed from the physical hatha yoga, but, on closer inspection, we can see that the eightfold path is always at the core. Strong, body-centred styles of yoga like Iyengar, power yoga and anusara yoga, and spiritual styles closer to the Indian practice, such as kundalini and kriya yoga, show how broadly and changeably the concept of yoga can be used. But all of the styles have one thing in common: the person, with all his or her facets, is at the centre. Yoga is intended to improve self-awareness, deepen our understanding of our own bodies and spirits, and allow us to obtain clarity. Patanjali himself provided an answer to the question of what yoga is:

Yoga is an act of looking inwards that allows us to know ourselves with greater clarity.

"Yoga is the removal of the fluctuations of the mind." (Patanjali, Yoga Sutras 1.1)

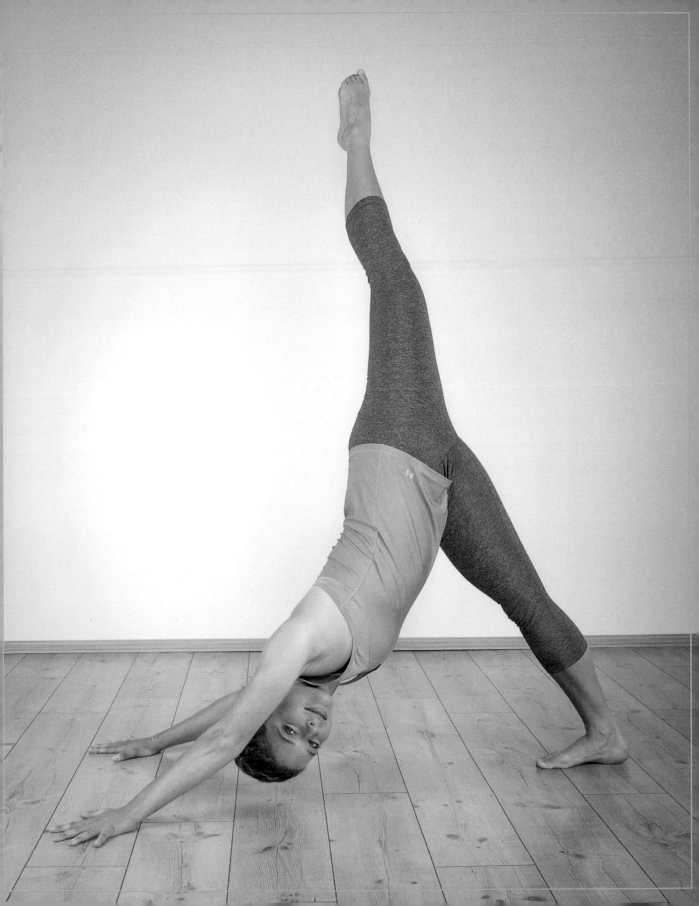

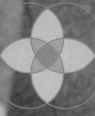

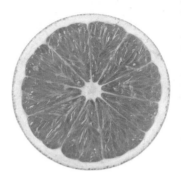

So what is this fascia we've been talking about? It is currently one of the most talked about tissues in sports science. Everybody is discussing it, and not only in the scientific world. Knowledge of the numerous functions of fascia enriches the worlds of both sport and yoga. But fascia has always been part of our bodies, it is nothing new! What are new are the recent insights from scientific studies which have enabled us to reconsider and expand on our ideas of our movement system. Until recently, we assumed that movements existed as a result of interactions between muscles, bones and the nervous system alone. While this is by no means false, we can now complement this view with another important component that greatly affects our movement system: fascia.

The term "fascia" covers all connective structures in the body.

Fascial tissues include:
» ligaments

» tendons

» aponeuroses

» subcutaneous tissue

» visceral fascia (covering the organs)

» neural fascia.

Muscles, bones, nerves and organs are all covered by fascia. Fascia connects everything in our body, and at the same time keeps everything separate. It is the link between external and internal body structures. And the best part? Fascia can be trained! So you can take action to ensure a healthy, flexible fascial network.

The structure of fascia
What does fascia have to do with oranges?
No, we are not talking about the "orange peel" –

otherwise known as cellulite – that can form as a result of weak connective tissues. Instead, I want you to imagine the cross-section of a freshly cut orange – it's the perfect way to explain fascia. The fruit is surrounded by white threads, that provide shape and stability. A cross-section of your body would look similar. The white fibres can be found throughout the body, and they surround all the anatomical organs. Each organ, nerve, blood vessel, muscle and muscle fibre is surrounded by fascia. Fascia also penetrates the structures, in order to provide organs and vessels with protection.

 It is incorrect to talk about fascia in the plural. We only have one large fascia, which connects everything together.

Ground substance
All the fascia cells and fibres are found in a liquid ground substance. This is like a big swimming pool, in which the cells and fibres are packed tightly together. The ground substance is mostly water, and it plays a major role as a shock absorber, for example in the case of impacts.

Fibres
The connective-tissue fibres in the fascia include collagen and elastin fibres. The amount and combination depends on the type of fascia. Collagen fibres make up the majority of the connective tissue fibres, being 60 to 70 percent. Collagen is a very firm structural protein and provides stability. You could compare collagen fibres to an almost unbreakable

The shaping organ

Fascia is the organ that gives us shape. If a disease were to remove everything but fascia from the human body, our shape would remain, despite having no muscles or bones.

Cells (metabolism)

Ground substance
(malleability and suppleness)

Fibres (mechanics)

Essentially, fascia comprise three components: the ground substance, fibres and cells.

rope. Elastin, the counterpart to collagen, is an elastic structural protein. In contrast to collagen fibres, elastin fibres are flexible and can be stretched by up to 100 to 150 percent! They act as a buffer for strain from stretching, and distribute the forces exerted evenly to the collagen. The two types of fibre have clear differences in terms of their structure. But they work together, hand in hand. An even balance between firm and elastic, hard and soft, is the basis for a healthy fascial network.

Cells

The cells in connective tissues are responsible for the metabolism of fascia. They produce the collagen and elastin, and are stimulated by movement. They react to the pulling and tension of stretching or springing movements by producing collagen or elastin.

Depending on the needs of the body, fascia can be taut, firm tissue (like the Achilles tendon) or loose connective tissue (for example the visceral fascia surrounding the organs).

Taut fascial tissue

The Achilles tendon is a perfect example. These tissues must withstand high tensile loads. The proportion of collagen is much higher than that of elastin. Tensile forces primarily act in two directions, up and down. The collagen fibres adapt their direction according to the tensile load. They are closely aligned and run parallel to each other in order to counterbalance the forces, like a strong steel cable.

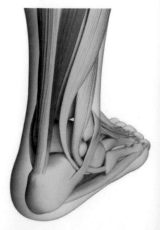

Loose fascial tissue

Let's take the liver as an example. It is surrounded by a fascial "cover" that separates it from other organs but connects it to them at the same time. The fibres here are arranged more freely and can move around. The proportion of water in the ground substance must be high, so that impacts and compressive loads are properly absorbed, and the organ is not damaged.

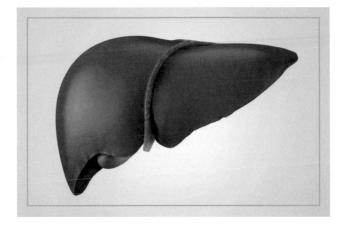

Fascia functions

The functions of fascia are just as varied as its manifestations:

» Connecting and separating: the fascial network is the only part of the body that connects all body parts together, while keeping tissues separate from each other at the same time.
» Support: without fascia, the musculoskeletal system wouldn't work, as it would have no stability (see page 19).
» Protection: all the pulling and tension our bodies are subjected to every day are buffered by fascia. The water in the ground substance and the fat cells are particularly important in this respect.
» Transferring forces: muscles and fascia are an inseparable unit. Fascia covers each individual muscle fibre, the muscle fibre bundles and the muscle as a whole. The muscle is attached to the bone with tendons. This means there is a permanent fascial connection to all structures needed for the mechanical transfer of forces.
» Transport: the ground substance plays an important role in metabolic processes, as nutrients and information from the blood and lymph vessels and the nerves are transported through it.

The body's pathway – fascial chains

Fascia forms an inseparable, interconnected unit. Nevertheless, fascial tissues can be roughly divided into three categories:

» Central nervous system fascia
» Organ fascia
» Musculoskeletal fascia.

Musculoskeletal fascia is particularly important for yoga, as it transfers forces and coordinates movement. The idea that bones are moved by the force of individual muscles and the muscular force is therefore transferred to the bone via one isolated tendon must be revised given what we now know about fascia. Fascia, which provides the "missing link", works hand in hand with muscles when it comes to transferring forces. Pulling and tension, as occur in stretching, are transferred from one part of the body to the next, so that the stress is distributed over the whole body.

The musculoskeletal fascia is also called "myofascia". The word myofascia describes the inseparable, interconnected unit of muscular tissue (myo-) and the connective fascial tissue (fascia). These chains are also often referred to as myofascial meridians, but chains to avoid confusion. The chains of the myofascial pathways are not acupuncture meridians, as meridians are usually understood as the energetic transmission lines in acupuncture. There are clear overlaps, but these two things are not synonymous.

Considering our body as a unit allows a holistic approach to finding the root of posture issues. Posture issues, such as a pronounced curving of the upper back ("hunchback"), lead to an imbalance between the front and back fascial chains: they are shortened on one side, and excessively stretched on the other. The body tries to compensate for this imbalance with chronic muscle tension. The fascia also contracts and thickens.

In fascia yoga, the pathways through our body provide a wonderful guiding principle for categorising poses. Think of this classification like a "body map" that helps you understand the effects of stretching and the distribution of forces. The following pathways are distinguished in fascia yoga:

» Back fascial chain
» Front fascial chain
» Side fascial chain
» Spiral fascial chain
» Arm chains.

Depending on the pathway, different effects will be obtained by stretching and activating the body:

Back fascial chain:
» Grounding of the feet and legs on the mat
» Upright and stable posture.

Front fascial chain:
» Opening the front chest for breathing deeply and freely
» Resolving anxious and protective postures.

Side fascial chains:
» Opening the side body to spread the lungs
» Stabilising the side body.

Spiral fascial chains:
» Stable stance (looping around the whole sole of the foot)
» Relaxing the neck and shoulder area (looping around the shoulder blades).

Arm chains:
» Stability in arm balances
» Opening the chest
» Relaxing the shoulders.

If you include exercises for all fascial chains in your practice, you can truly experience your whole body. Perhaps you will notice that the exercises for one fascial chain are easier for you than others. Be mindful and observe these differences. This will help you to find any imbalances in your body.

What does healthy fascia look like?
Everything you have learned about fascia so far makes it clear how much of an impact healthy, flexible fascia can have on the body. Healthy fascia can be described as:

» smooth
» watery
» elastic
» resilient
» slippery.

It has a healthy balance between smoothness and stability, and is elastic and resilient to tears. It absorbs pressure and impacts, but withstands high tensile loads at the same time.

It is possible to derive training methods from this alone. Pressing the tissue with the fascia roller helps improve hydration (water content). Springing, bouncing and jumping keep fascia elastic and resistant. Stretching gives smoothness.

This balance I describe is, of course, the ideal state, but only exists in the rarest cases. Your body, and your highly intelligent fascial tissues, have to adjust to everyday wear and tear. Too much or too little use leads to changes in the balance. Lots of sitting can lead to a loss in suppleness and elasticity, and at some point, the different parts of the fascia found throughout the body are no longer watery enough to slide over each other easily. The consequences of this range from muscle tension to painful stuck joints.

However, a lack of movement is not always at the root of these issues. Too much stress, through sport or one-sided activity, can also damage the fascial network. As you have already read, the cells in fascia are stimulated by movement to create collagen fibres that then align themselves as needed. In itself, this is a good thing, as long as it is done in moderation. Constant, unchanged movement, however, will lead to too much collagen being produced at specific sites in the body. Collagen is the resistant steel-cable type of fascial fibre. Gradually, you will find that your body loses mobility in these areas.

Fascia training shouldn't be restricted to your yoga mat. Fascia likes to move – in lots of different ways! Make sure your daily routine is full of movement and variety.

Practice
Now you know more about fascia and the specificities of fascia yoga, it's time to put this into practice! I'm sure you are looking forward to experiencing how the theoretical fascial model applies to your body. So here are a few general tips before you start your practice. In the following catalogue of exercises, one petal of the fascia yoga flower is always the focus. They include familiar yoga exercises and many fascial variations.

Chapter 3

On the mat - From theory to practice

The two previous chapters explained fascia as a part of the body, and the specificities of fascia yoga. With these foundations in place, it's time to practise! I'm sure you are looking forward to experiencing how the theoretical fascial model applies to your body.

How to use the catalogue of exercises

You have already learned about the five training elements in fascia yoga using the fascia yoga flower. Each of the petals is presented in its own chapter, with a short theoretical introduction and an extensive practical part. You will learn everything you need to know on the individual exercises and what in particular you should pay attention to. Chapter 9 brings together elements of the preceding five chapters. I have put together special fascia yoga practices for different focal points and levels of difficulty. This includes the fascia salutation, a "fascial modification" to the sun salutation.

But before you get started with the catalogue of exercises, I recommend going through the basics, such as posture, hand and foot work, and starting positions, in theory and practice. Think of this chapter as a handy reference work for the correct alignment of your body.

Spine and pelvis – our focal point

The spine

Our spinal column – or, more accurately, our spinal chain, as it's certainly not a rigid column – is as a whole a very mobile structure, made up of vertebrae and joints that are moved by a complex system of muscle and fascia. Our spine has seven cervical vertebrae, twelve thoracic vertebrae and five lumbar vertebrae, as well as the sacrum and the coccyx. A healthy, normally aligned spine has a double-S-shaped curve. The cervical spine and lumbar spine both curve towards the front of the body (described as a lordotic curve). The thoracic spine, sacrum and coccyx curve towards the

back of the body (known as a kyphotic curve). If these curves are too strong or too weak, this leads to poor posture, which can have an effect on the surrounding joints (shoulders, pelvis, etc.). To combat this poor posture, we need the right level of tension in the body.

The S-shaped curve of the back of the body generally continues above and below the spine (skull, hollows of the knees). Our whole body is aligned according to this principle in order to best absorb external forces.

Our spine controls the movements of the joints in our bodies. It can:

» move them forwards and backwards (flexing and extending)
» move them around an axis (rotating)
» tilt them sideways (lateral flexing)
» lengthen them.

The last takes place before the three other types of movement. Whether you are moving a joint forwards (flexion), backwards (extension), sideways (lateral flexion) or around (rotation), you first create space and length in the spine in order to carry out the movement in alignment, with a healthy double-S shape.

The pelvis

While we are talking about the spine, we should also mention the pelvis. The pelvis and spine are one unit, dynamically connected to each other. Think of the pelvis as the base of the spine. Figuratively speaking, the pelvis is like a vase and the spine a flower standing in it. If you want to move the flower from A to B, where do you hold? That's right, the vase! And it's the same with the spine. If you want to move your spine, it makes sense to start the movement from your pelvis.

As an example, here's a quick and easy exercise:

Pelvic tilt

Tilt your pelvis forwards and backwards a few times. Try both ways! Then tilt your pelvis forwards and come into a forward fold. Observe how it feels in your spine, and how far your can lean forwards. Then repeat with your pelvis tilted backwards. Can you feel a difference? If you want to bring your spine into a forward fold, tilt your pelvis forward. The spine follows the movement of the pelvis and also moves forward. The pelvis and the spine work together, not against each other. If you are in forward fold and don't feel a pull in the backs of your legs, you can straighten your knees. However, when folding forward from the pelvis, in terms of your anatomy it is sensible to bend your knees. This will eliminate the direct tensile load, which in turn gives the pelvis more mobility.

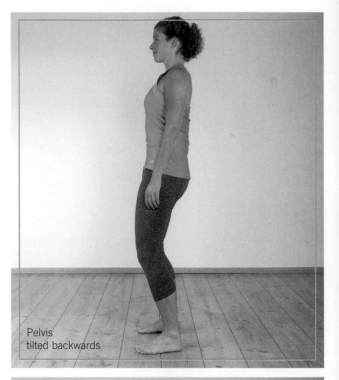

Pelvis
tilted backwards

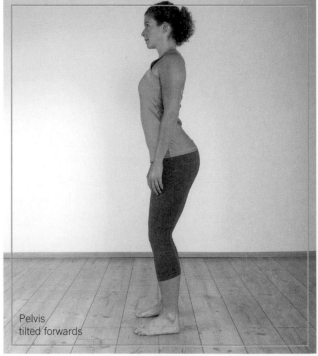

Pelvis
tilted forwards

Tensegrity in yoga

The tensegrity model comes from architecture, and serves as an example for self-stabilising structures. Initially it may seem strange to try to explain the human body using an architectural model, but essentially, it is just that. Tensegrity combines tension and integrity. Our body is a unit that requires tension in order to maintain its integrity. In this model, the struts are bones, the elastic bands are fascia, and the junctions are joints.

Each part has a role to play. If we change something in one place – for example moving a joint – this movement has an effect on the whole system. In exactly the same way, tensions in the fascial system can lead to the position of a joint being changed. This results in poor posture and imbalances, as our body is always trying to bring the whole structure back into place. Our body is not a two-dimensional system built of blocks, like a wall. The whole structure balances the stresses that gravity, powerful stretching and impacts can cause. Consequently, our head is not just held up by the uppermost cervical vertebra, but by the whole body. And the lumbar vertebrae don't have to carry the whole weight of the spine. The whole network contributes.

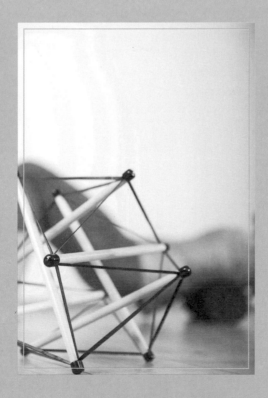

Hand and foot work in yoga – for a healthy practice

Hands

In all arm balances, the hands are the foundations of the body. We usually keep the feet, or at least one foot, on the mat. Exercises like the handstand place a great deal of strain on the hands and wrists. To ensure you can continue leaning on them for a long time, don't forget the following:

» Place the hands flat and wide.
» The fingers should be spread widely, but with the thumbs sticking out roughly two-thirds of the way.
» The middle and index fingers are parallel to each other, in line with the shoulders.
» Think of your palm as a square and try to press all four corners of the square into the mat.
» Press the fingertips firmly into the mat.

In yoga, this planting of the hands is also called hasta bandha. It is the starting point for stabilising and activating the arms and shoulders when the weight is primarily supported by the hands in arm balances.

Feet

The feet are our foundation in many yoga postures. They are our connection to the mat, and often support our whole body. We should really pay more attention to our feet – and not just on the mat! They play a supporting role – in the truest sense of the term! – in our lives and on the yoga mat. You develop a stable base for the whole body from the feet up. For a sturdy, upright posture when standing on one or both feet, don't forget these important points:

» Spread your weight evenly over all four corners of the feet. Root the heels, the balls of the feet, and the inner and outer edges evenly into the mat.
» Spread the toes apart.
» Consciously push the big toe and the little toe into the mat, without clawing them. This activates the arch of the foot, lifting it upwards.

Rooting through the feet is called pada bandha. This provides a straight posture for the whole body in all standing poses and balances.

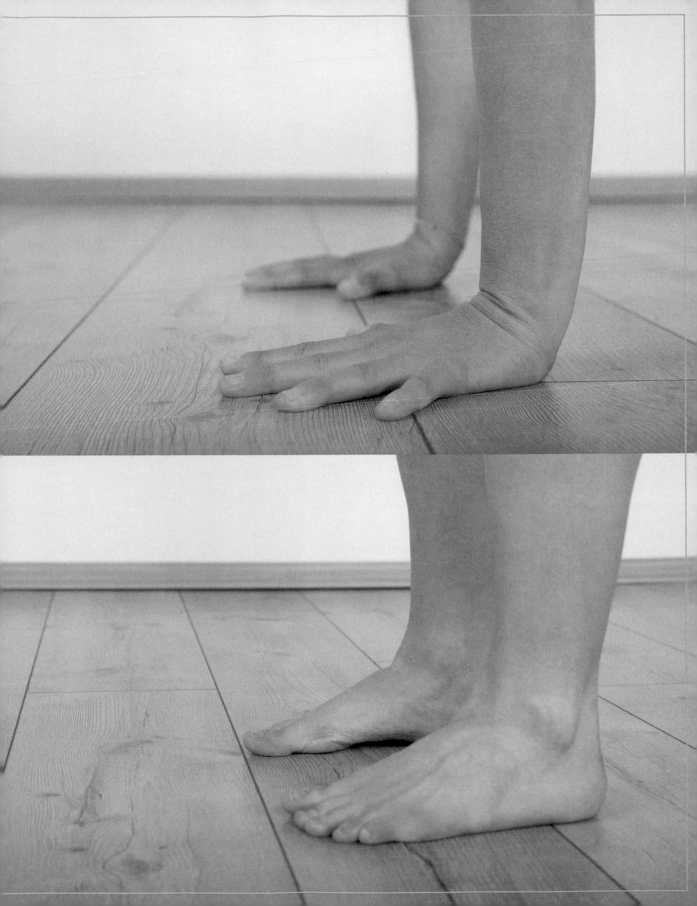

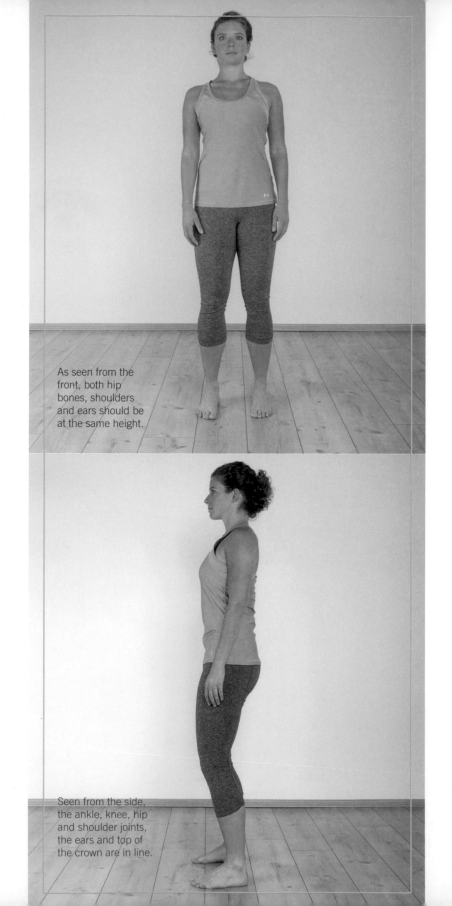

As seen from the
front, both hip
bones, shoulders
and ears should be
at the same height.

Seen from the side,
the ankle, knee, hip
and shoulder joints,
the ears and top of
the crown are in line.

Starting positions

If we have the right starting position for each exercise, we are already halfway to a healthy, beneficial practice. When the foundations are right, you will find the exercises easier. As you do the exercises from the catalogue, you'll notice that the starting positions are often the same. The following poses are the foundations for proper alignment and posture during your practice.

Standing position

A consciously aligned, straight position relieves the joints and provides stability and steadiness. Practise this pose for a few minutes and you'll discover how complex standing can be!

» Place your feet parallel, hip width apart. Root evenly into the mat with both feet (see page 22).
» As seen from the front, both hip bones, shoulders and ears should be at the same height.

» The knees are straight. Activate your thigh muscles. This will raise your kneecaps slightly, ensuring the knees are not overstretched.
» Activate your abdominal muscles slightly and tuck your tailbone downwards.
» Lift your breastbone forwards and upwards, gently sliding the shoulders back and down.
» The arms rest at the sides of the body.
» Look forwards into the distance.
» Imagine that an invisible thread is pulling the back of your head upwards, lengthening the neck.

Go through all of the alignment points again, from bottom to top. If you are new to the practice and are not sure whether your body is aligned symmetrically, practise in front of a mirror.

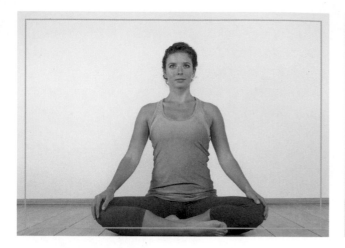

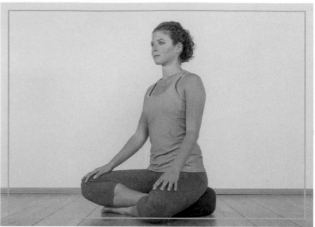

Cross-legged position

The upright sitting posture is the original yoga pose, taken from the oldest traditions. It is a symbol for meditation, calm and stillness. A lack of mobility in the hips and spine often means that sitting for long periods can be uncomfortable and difficult. Find the right sitting position for you.

» Sit down and cross your legs. If you like, place the heels under the thighs.
» Feel your sitting bones, and root them into the mat or cushion.
» Align your pelvis. The spine follows this alignment.
» Lift your breastbone forwards and upwards, gently sliding the shoulders back and down.
» Let your pelvis sink into the floor and, at the same time, imagine an invisible thread pulling the back of your head upwards, lengthening the neck. This lengthens the spine, working against gravity, and relieves pressure on the intervertebral discs.

Tip: For proper alignment of the pelvis and spine, t is important that the knees are lower than the hips. Use a cushion or blanket, or roll up your mat, in order to sit higher. Try several heights to find the right one for you.

 I recommend practising yoga barefoot. This allows you to feel a direct connection with the mat. You see your feet and, if you hold your feet, you can better feel the contact. In addition, your toes can work better, and you have a much stronger grip on the mat. Try it out!

Kneeling pose

Kneeling pose is an alternative to cross-legged position. In fascia yoga, it is used as the starting position for back bends and side bends.

» Sit on your lower legs and feet. The tops of the feet are flat, and the buttocks lie on the heels. The thighs remain parallel.

» Align your spine so that the lower back is straight.
» The breastbone lifts up and the shoulders slide down the back so that the neck is long and relaxed.

When seen from the side, the hips and shoulders are aligned.

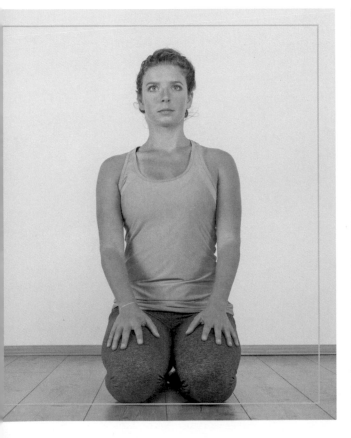
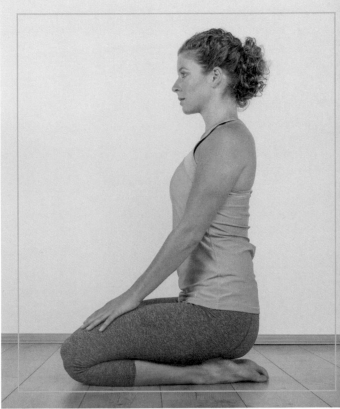

Tabletop position

Tabletop position is one of the most common starting positions for arm balances. It provides a good position for practising aligning the hands.

» Place the hands directly under the shoulders and the knees under the hips. Lay the tops of the feet on the mat.
» Align the hands so that they are spread widely and rooted into the mat (hasta bandha; see page 20).
» Bend the elbows very slightly.
» Consciously pull the shoulders away from the ears. This lengthens the neck.
» Direct your gaze to the floor, so that the head is aligned with the cervical spine.
» Imagine that an invisible thread is pulling the crown of your head forwards and your tailbone backwards.

High lunge

High lunge stretches the hip flexors. It creates a stable foundation for many standing poses.

» Start in tabletop position and move the right leg forwards between the hands. The ankle and knee are aligned.
» Stretch your left leg backwards.
» Activate the thigh muscles in your left leg and stretch the hollow of the knee towards the ceiling.
» The pelvis is lowered.
» Lift your upper body a little. Move onto your fingertips and lengthen the spine by lifting your heart centre forwards.
» Keep the head aligned with the cervical spine.

Downward-facing dog (see page 54) is also a good way to move into high lunge. From downward-facing dog, lift the right leg and place it between the hands. If your foot is not directly between the hands, grip your ankle and gently move the foot forwards.

Tip: Slide the right knee forwards a fraction, and push backwards into the left heel. You will feel a wonderful stretch through the body, and your legs will form a stable foundation. Moving the upper body will now be easier. A stable foundation creates freedom and ease in the upper body, giving you a greater range of motion.

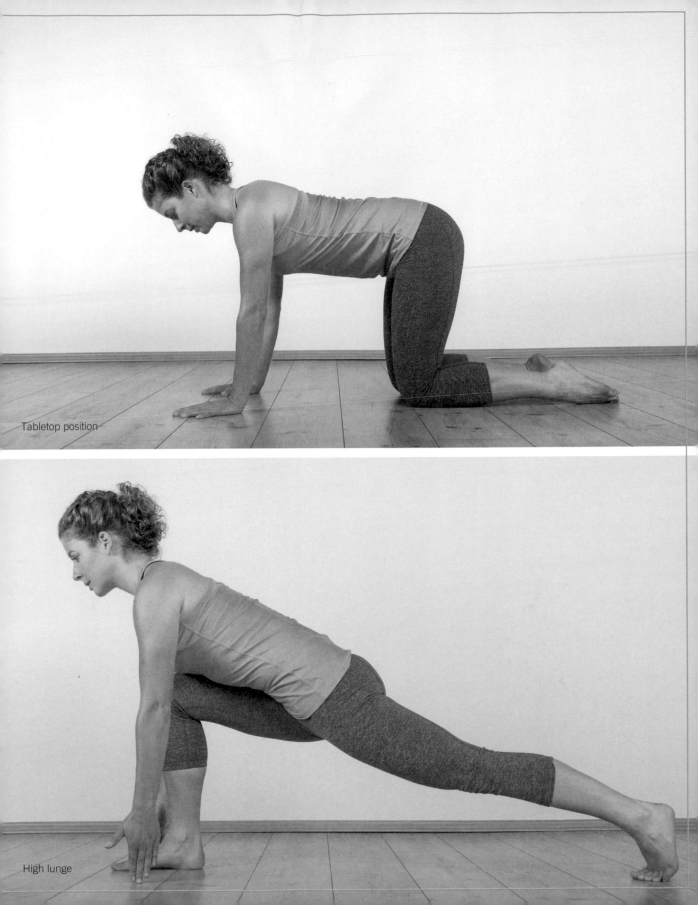

Tabletop position

High lunge

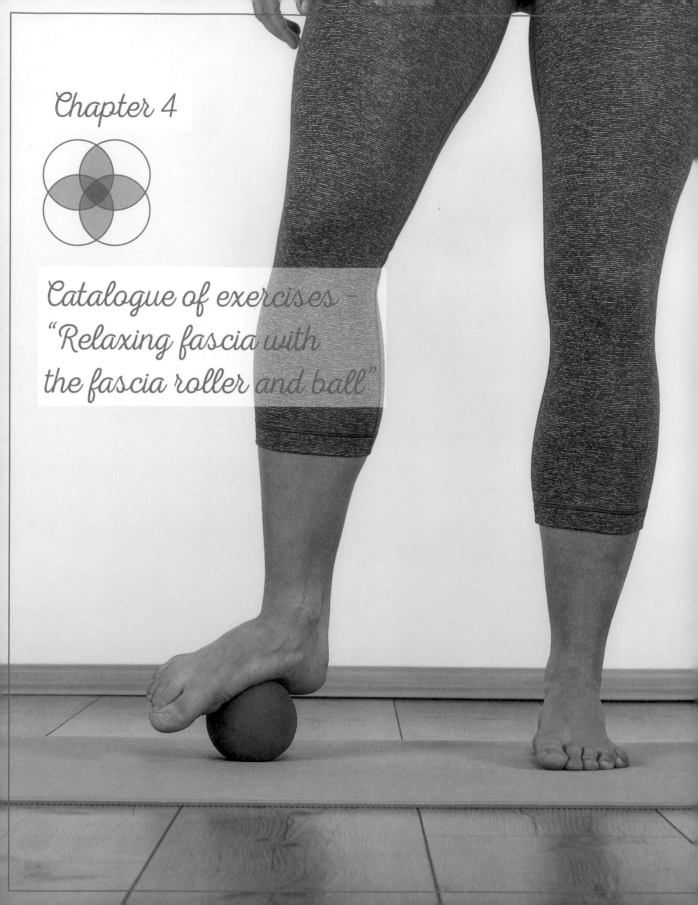

Chapter 4

Catalogue of exercises – "Relaxing fascia with the fascia roller and ball"

When the body is unbalanced

The body tends to adjust to its usual movement pattern. Overstressing the body, for example through intensive training or repetitive movements, leads to tensions. And this in turn leads to "stuck" fascia. But a lack of movement can also be a potential cause of loss of suppleness in the connective tissue. Painful tensions and stiffness are the result. So the key is to not let things get this far!

Why roll?

Rolling the connective tissues using a fascia roller and fascia ball has a similar effect on fascia as a massage. The aim of rolling is to press old, exhausted fluids out of the fascia, so that the tissues can be refilled with fresh fluids. Here, we are working with the ground substance in fascia. Figuratively, you can imagine that you are wringing out your connective tissues like a sponge, taking away metabolic waste products, toxins and lymphatic fluids. When the pressure is released, this sponge then refills with new fluids – so the fascial network remains properly hydrated and supple, and the layers can glide across each other with ease.

Right after you try it for the first time, you'll feel how warm, mobile and relaxed the rolled areas seem. This is thanks to the increased circulation and reduced tension in the muscles and fascia. The following exercises are therefore a wonderful introduction to your fascia yoga practice. They will help to keep your body supple and stimulated. This beneficial regenerative effect can also be used after a strong yoga session in order to reduce, or "roll out", the tension that has built up in the body

Beneficial effects of rolling:

» "Sticky" areas are released.
» Muscle tensions are reduced.
» Awareness of the body is increased.
» Pains and muscle soreness are reduced.
» Fluid supply is stimulated.

Ready, set, roll!

Now that you know why you should include rolling in your fascia yoga practice, the next question is how. There are a few things to bear in mind for an effective, beneficial roller experience.

» Rolling speed: I recommend slow, conscious rolling. Your breathing can be a good guide. One breath per centimetre is a perfect speed. Concentrate fully on the part of the body you want to reach, and give yourself time.
» Painful areas: You are certain to find areas that are more painful than others to roll, as they are more tense or "sticky". This is completely normal. Think of it as your body showing you where the roller is really needed! Don't just roll over these areas, but stay there for a few breaths, until the tissue softens and the pain subsides.
» Intensity: The intensity of the rolling depends on your subjective perception of pain. But don't think that the more painful, the better! Remember that fascia is full of pain receptors, and the goal is not to target them. Your breathing can be a good indicator here, too. If it is relaxed and even, you've found the right balance.

Which roller is right for me?

Choosing the right roller is key to the positive effect of fascia massage. A wide range of rollers and balls are available on the market, with various degrees of hardness, lengths, structures and diameters. Above all, the hardness, or firmness, of the roller is key. Each person has to make an individual decision on what is best for him or her. In principle, the roller should be softer rather than too hard, ensuring the pleasant "good pain" sensation when rolling slowly, as described above. Soft products like Pilates rollers, Franklin balls and tennis balls can also be helpful if you are particularly tense.

The diameter of the roller influences the "roller feeling". The bigger the diameter, the larger the pressure distribution. This means less discomfort is felt. And the same applies for balls. You can work larger areas with a large ball, or go deeper into the tissue with a small ball. Investing in a ball – or even using a simple tennis ball – is definitely worthwhile. You can reach targeted problem areas, and roll them out selectively and intensively.

Small, light, cheap

Fascia rollers can be bought for as little as £20, while fascia balls are available for £10 to £15. A tennis ball also does the job, although it loses firmness over time, so it is worth buying a fascia ball. Rollers and balls are light and don't take up much space, so they are easy to take with you when you're on the go. They can be bought online, but also in specialist orthopaedics shops and sports shops.

Catalogue of exercises

The following catalogue of exercises moves through the body gradually, from the soles of your feet (plantar fascia) to your neck muscles.

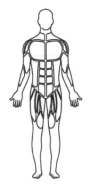

Soles of the feet

The fascia in the soles of the feet – the plantar fascia – runs from the balls of the feet to the heels, moving into the Achilles tendon. It is the lowest part of the back fascial chain (see chapter 2).

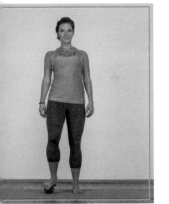

You need: Fascia ball or tennis ball
Start in a standing position. Place your right heel on the ball and slowly roll the foot over the ball towards the toes. When you arrive at the toe joints, roll the ball under the arch and towards the outer edge of the foot. Explore and feel the whole sole of your foot, allowing the ball to slowly melt into the tissue. Start with little pressure, and increase gradually.

You will feel some areas more intensely. Stay in these areas for a moment (30 to 60 seconds), and you will see that these tense areas gradually disappear with time. Once you've felt this release, continue to explore the sole of your foot. Take two to three minutes for your right foot, then change to the left.

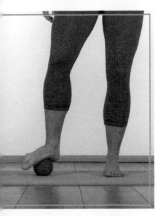

Benefits for your yoga practice
Rolling the plantar fascia is one of the easiest and most effective exercises in this book, and should be a part of every fascia yoga practice. It helps the sensory activation of your foundations, supports centring, and promotes the connection between your body and the mat. This means that the exercise is a wonderful way to prepare for all standing poses – in particular, balances. Rolling the soles of the feet is also recommended before forward bends, as it stimulates the back fascial chain.

Notes: If a tennis ball or fascia ball is not firm enough for you, you can also roll the soles of the feet with a golf ball. This is a much more targeted approach. You can vary the pressure yourself by shifting your body weight.

Mobility self-assessment

Before rolling the soles of the feet

Stand upright, with your feet hip width apart. Roll downwards, vertebra by vertebra, until you can't move any further downwards. If your fingertips don't touch the ground, take note of the distance between your fingertips and the ground. If you can reach the ground easily, take note of the current stretch in the backs of your legs. Now roll the soles of the feet as described on page 31.

After rolling the soles of the feet

Repeat the exercise, rolling your upper body down towards the floor as described above. Can you reach further this time? Has the distance between your fingertips and the ground decreased? If you could already touch the ground on your first try, compare how the backs of your legs feel now, after working the soles of the feet.

Try it out!

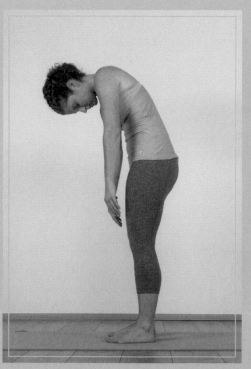

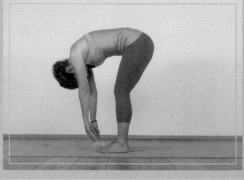

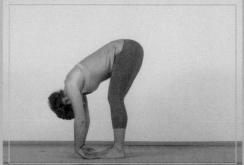

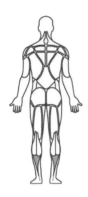

Achilles tendon

The Achilles tendon is the thickest, strongest tendon in the body, and has to withstand huge pressures. It acts as a transition between the calf muscles and the heel. It doesn't simply start or stop at the heel bone, but provides a direct connection to the plantar fascia, forming an important force-transmitting part of the back fascial chain.

You need: Fascia roller
Sit on the floor with your legs out straight in front of you, and place the roller under the Achilles tendon of your right leg – between the calf muscle and the heel. Support yourself on your hands, placed around one hand's width behind your buttocks, lift your breastbone and slide your shoulders down your back. Cross the left leg over the right, and begin to slowly circle the right foot as it lies on the roller. Change directions after approximately 30 seconds. Finally, repeat this exercise on the other side.

Benefits for your yoga practice
The Achilles tendon is part of the back fascial chain and in many forward bends acts as a transfer point for forces between the calf and foot muscles. In poses like downward-facing dog, forward fold and warrior, there is a strong tensile stress on the calf muscles, which – as everything in our body is interconnected – is primarily transmitted to the Achilles tendon. Circling the Achilles tendon on the fascia roller supports the smooth sliding of the tendon structure and keeps it supple and mobile.

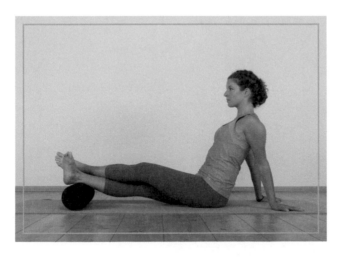

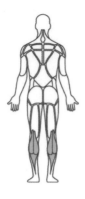

Calves

The calf muscles are also part of the back fascial chain and comprise three main muscles. They provide a connection between the ankle and knee joints. In terms of function, the calf muscles move when the knee joint is flexed and the ankle joint is rotated externally.

You need: Fascia roller
Sit on the floor with your legs out straight in front of you, and place the roller under your left calf. Place your right foot next to the left knee. Support yourself on your hands, placed around one hand's width behind your buttocks, and lift the buttocks. Roll along the length of the calf. To do this, slide your body forward from the shoulders in order to reach all of the area between the hollow of the knee and the Achilles tendon. After approximately one minute, sit back on the floor and change to the other side.

Variation 1: Place the roller under the right calf. Now cross the left leg over the right in order to increase the intensity.

Variation 2: You can also vary the movement. The gastrocnemius muscle – the two-headed calf muscle – gives the calf its shape. While rolling, move the toes inwards and outwards in order to reach both parts of the muscle.

Note: Rolling the calves can often be very intensive. Take particular care to maintain quiet, flowing breathing. Begin with the gentle variation with less pressure.

Benefits for your yoga practice
Rolling the calves is particularly recommended before forward bends. The calf area is generally rather tense and contracted, which limits the range of motion in forward bends. But all of the muscles in the back of the lower leg are also active in standing poses. Rolling activates the sensory receptors and sensitises the muscle–fascia system.

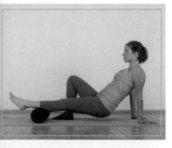

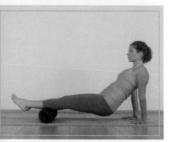

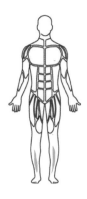

Shins

The muscles in the front of the lower leg include the extensors, found to the sides. They extend the big and little toes and the ankle joint.

You need: Fascia roller
Come into tabletop position (see page 26) and place the roller in front of your knees. Move the left leg forward and place the lower leg below the knee on the roller. Tilt your buttocks to the left in order to protect the shin bone, so that only the outer edge of the lower leg lies on the roller. Now slowly roll the shin from the ankle joint to just under the knee. After approximately one minute, change to the other leg.

Note: Make sure that the foot remains relaxed and there is no muscle tension in the area being rolled.

Benefits for your yoga practice
In all standing poses and balances, the muscle–fascia network in the lower leg plays an important stabilising role. The front and back of the lower leg work together, not against each other, as they are connected by the major lower-leg fascia – the crural fascia. Rolling the calves and shins is good preparation for all standing poses and particularly for balances.

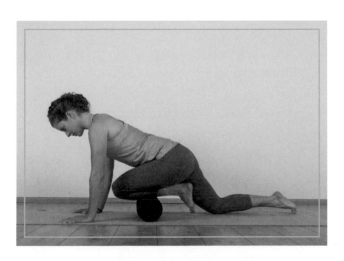

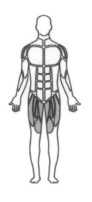

Thighs

The four-headed thigh muscle (quadriceps femoris) forms the front of the upper part of the leg. It comprises four muscle portions that are responsible for extending the knee. The four muscle portions converge into one tendon, which runs over the kneecap to the lower leg. This part of the muscle is to a large extent responsible for stabilising the knee joint. Furthermore, other parts of the thigh muscle are also responsible for moving the hips.

You need: Fascia roller
Kneel on the mat and place the roller in front of your knees. Come into a forearm balance, so that the thighs rest on the roller. Activate your abdominal muscles and pull the shoulders away from the ears. Your body forms a line parallel to the floor. Slide your whole body backwards from the shoulders and roll your thighs to just below the hips. Finally, roll back to just above the knees. Continue this slow rolling for one to two minutes.

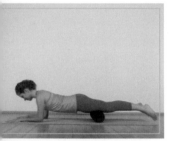

Tip: Vary the movement by turning your toes in and out while rolling in order to reach all areas of the thighs.

Note: Maintain tension in your buttocks so that your body remains parallel to the floor.

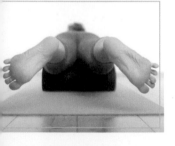

Benefits for your yoga practice

The thighs are part of the front fascial chain. They are involved in all back bends, as parts of the large thigh muscle are responsible for moving the hips. Rolling these parts makes this naturally firm area softer, and makes it easier to extend the hips. Rolling this area is recommended for intensive back bends with strong stretching through the hips, such as wheel and camel pose.

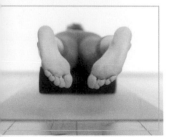

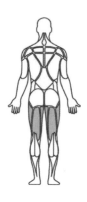

Hamstrings

The hamstring muscles, at the back of the thigh, are also called the ischiocrural muscles. They are the counterparts to the front thigh muscles. They run from the ischial tuberosity (the sitting bones) down to the lower leg and protect the knee from behind. They have two main functions: hip extension and knee flexion.

You need: Fascia roller

Sit on the mat with your legs out in front of you. Place the roller under your hamstrings, just behind the hollows of the knees. Support yourself on your hands behind your buttocks and lift the buttocks. Now slide your body forwards from the shoulders. Slowly roll your whole hamstring area. When you arrive at the buttocks, roll back to the starting position. Roll in both directions for around one minute.

Tip: The supporting positions for rolling the legs mean that you may feel some discomfort in your arms and wrists. In between exercises, rest on your buttocks and relax the arms, wrists and shoulders. Then start again, slowly increasing the intensity to be able to hold the supporting position for longer periods.

Benefits for your yoga practice

A lack of mobility in the hamstrings and hips can be a limiting factor when it comes to forward bends. Make sure to roll the full length of the hamstrings, so that you also reach the muscle–tendon connections in the hollow of the knee. This makes it easier for you to keep your knees straight in a forward bend. By rolling the hamstrings up to the buttocks, you reach the muscles that allow the hips to extend and have a direct impact on the mobility of the hips.

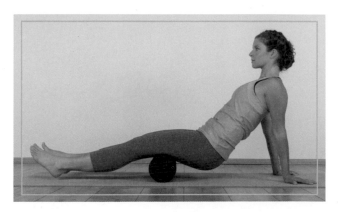

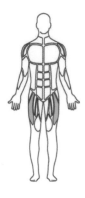

Outer thighs

The muscles in the outer thighs are covered by the fascia lata. This part of the fascia is put under heavy strain, as it connects the hip area to the knee and stabilises the leg for everyday movements like walking.

You need: Fascia roller
Lie on your left side, supported by your arm, and place the roller under the left outer thigh. Your left leg remains straight and relaxed. The right leg and upper arm serve to support the body. Roll the outer thigh slowly between the knee and hip. After approximately one minute, change to the other side.

Note: Make sure to keep the supporting shoulder stable.

Tip: Don't be surprised if rolling certain areas of the outer thigh is more painful than relaxing at first! The fascia lata is large and is put under a lot of stress in everyday life. Spend time consciously rolling the most painful areas, as that is where your body needs it most. A variation using the fascia ball or a tennis ball on the wall is particularly useful here. You can reach the affected area in a targeted, specific way. Roll the tense areas in slow, circling movements. Vary the pressure and direction of the rolling.

Benefits for your yoga practice
By rolling the outer thigh, you work both the lateral and spiral fascial chains. In yoga, this is particularly good preparation for side bends and twists.

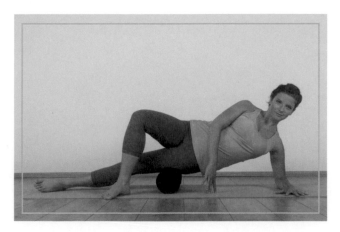

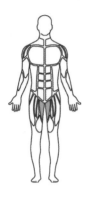

Inner thighs

The muscle group along the inner thigh, the adductors, moves the legs towards the centre of the body. For example, moving a splayed leg back in. The adductors run from the pubic bone down to the thigh bone.

You need: Fascia roller
Lie on your stomach, supporting yourself on your forearms. Place the roller parallel to your body, about level with your left hip. Bend your left leg to the side and lay the upper thigh on the roller. Now slowly roll the inner thigh from the groin to just under the knee. After approximately one minute, change to the other side.

Variation: This is more intensive with a fascia ball or tennis ball. The starting position and exercise are identical. You simply place the fascia ball between the floor and your inner thigh, and move the thigh up and down or in circles from the hip. The smaller surface area means you should feel more pressure, and can roll painful areas in a more targeted way.

Tip: Breath into the relaxation. Stay at any tense areas and let the ball melt into the zone. Breath deeply three or four times. With each exhalation, your thigh sinks more deeply into the ball.

Benefits for your yoga practice
Massaging the inner thigh prepares the muscle–fascia network for hip-opening poses. A supple inner thigh will make poses like triangle and extended side angle easier.

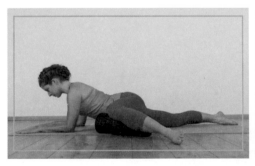 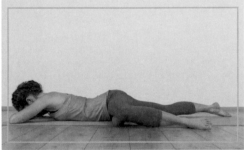

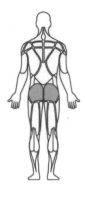

Buttocks

The gluteus maximus is our biggest muscle, and also one of the most powerful. It covers other, smaller muscles that lie underneath it. The key role of all the muscles in the buttocks is to extend the hips. They thus have a significant impact on our upright posture. Upwards, these muscles are directly connected to the lumbar fascia, the large area of fascia in the lower back. And downwards, there is a direct connection to the fascia lata – the strong band of fascia leading to the outer thigh.

You need: Fascia roller

Sit on the roller, with your feet on the floor. Support yourself with your hands on the floor behind you. Place your left foot on your right knee and shift your weight to the left side of your buttocks, so that only this side is in contact with the roller. Roll slowly forwards and backwards from the sitting bones to the lower back. After approximately one minute, change to the other side.

Variation: The exercise can be made more intensive with a fascia ball or tennis ball. Roll your buttocks slowly in circles over the fascia ball, making sure to reach the lateral areas.

Benefits for your yoga practice

Stuck, tense muscles in the buttocks can lead to pain in the lower back and significantly reduce the mobility of the hips as a result of poor posture in the pelvic area. Our hips are our focal point in everyday life and on the yoga mat (chapter 3). The muscles in the buttocks are the main element involved in extending the hips. Before hip-opening poses like cross-legged position, I recommend rolling the buttocks intensively.

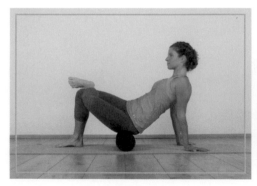
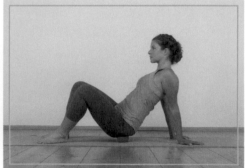

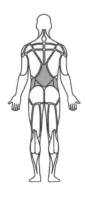

Lower back

Between the muscles of the back and the skin, there is a large diamond-shaped layer of fascia – the lumbar or thoracolumbar fascia. It connects the pelvis with the upper limbs and transfers forces in both directions. It surrounds the large back muscle and covers the whole lower back. It leads upwards along the spine to the bottom rib.

You need: Fascia roller
Sit on the floor with the feet placed flat, and place the roller directly behind your buttocks. Support yourself with your forearms placed behind you, and at the same time lift your buttocks off the floor. Roll yourself across the roller until it is placed directly under the lumbar spine area. Slowly roll this area. Keep active tension in the abdominal muscles, and the head in line with the cervical spine.

Note: The lumbar spine is made up of only five vertebrae. The surface rolled during this exercise measures approximately 5–10 cm. Make sure that you stay within this area.

Benefits for your yoga practice
Almost all yoga poses require and promote the mobility and stability of the spine. Forward bends, back bends, twists, side bends and balances – they all make the spine move in different ways. The lumbar fascia is stretched in forward bends. Rolling this part of the back fascial chain promotes suppleness and allows you to fold further and more easily.

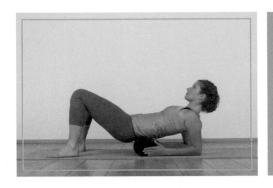

Scientists have observed that the lumbar fascia in patients with chronic back pain is much thicker and firmer than in patients with no pain. Furthermore, researchers investigating fascia have found that there are many pain receptors in the lumbar fascia. This means that when dealing with back pain, it is important to take the fascia into consideration, not only the intervertebral discs.

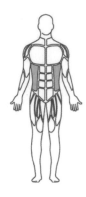

Side body

The "side body" muscles include the inner and outer lateral abdominal muscles and the transverse abdominals. They are directly connected to the back fascia.

You need: Fascia roller
Lie on your side, supporting yourself on your forearm. Move your top leg forward to add support. Place the roller under your waist and lie on it. Gently, with very little pressure at first, roll the side body from the hip to the ribs.

Make sure that your pelvis stays straight and doesn't twist upwards or downwards. Your rolling should be as straight as possible. After approximately one minute, change to the other side.

Note: During the exercise, make sure you maintain flowing, relaxed breathing.

Benefits for your yoga practice
Rolling the side body is particularly recommended before side bends and twists. You primarily reach the side fascial chain, which is involved in the lateral movement of the body, amongst other things. The side chain also serves as a "brake" for twists. Rolling can also increase the range of motion for twists.

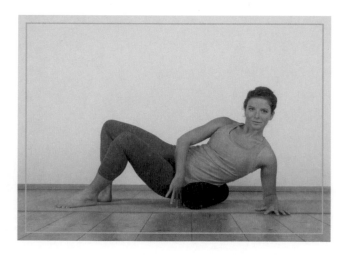

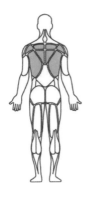

Upper back

The thoracic area comprises twelve vertebrae, and therefore has a much greater surface area than the lumbar spine. The thoracic spine curves backwards slightly (kyphotic curve). This corresponds to the spine's natural S shape. However, in many people, our everyday movement patterns (for example sitting at a desk) substantially intensify this curve.

You need: Fascia roller
Sit on the floor with your feet placed flat, and place the roller around 20–30 cm behind you on the mat. Lean backwards over the roller and lift your buttocks off the mat. Cross your arms over your chest. Keep the abdominal muscles active. Roll the area between the shoulder blades and the lower back for approximately one minute.

Then move both feet one step forward, so that the roller lies under the shoulder blades, and include this area in your rolling. Roll here for approximately one more minute.

Variation: You can open your chest further by interlocking your hands behind your head. Open the elbows outwards and slowly glide across the roller. By opening the chest, you can achieve a much greater stretch in the thoracic spine. Slowly experiment with opening the chest.

Benefits for your yoga practice
You will see that rolling this area makes the shoulders and chest much more flexible. This is particularly noticeable in back bends like cobra. In warrior, you will also find it easier to lift the heart centre. Twists are made easier as you also reach parts of the spiral fascial chain.

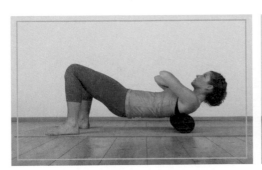
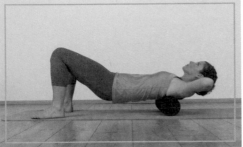

Standing back massage

You can use a fascia ball or tennis ball to really work tense parts of the back, as the ball can reach targeted areas the large surface of the roller can't. If you have specific painful tense areas, it can be helpful to work through these tensions while standing. Another advantage of the standing variation is the ability to adjust the pressure.

You need: Fascia ball or tennis ball

Stand with your back to the wall and place the ball to the side of your lumbar spine in the soft tissue. Press your body against the ball and wall. Start to roll the whole area with small circular movements. If you find a painful area, stay there with the ball for three to four deep breaths. With each exhalation, press your body a little further into the wall and with each inspiration, release the pressure again. Then change over to the other side of the spine. Take hold of the ball and move it to the other side. Don't roll over your vertebrae with the ball!

The lateral areas along the thoracic spine and shoulder blades can also be comfortably rolled in a standing position as described. This enables you to systematically observe where your body tends to be more or less tense. The areas in which these tensions occur vary greatly, and depend on the stresses your body is exposed to. It is completely normal to feel significant differences between the left and right sides of your body.

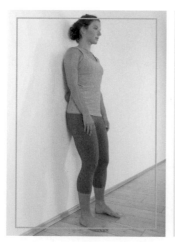 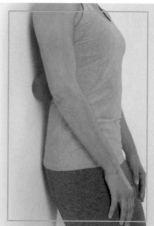 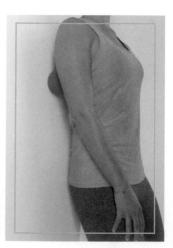

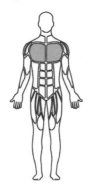

Chest

The large chest muscle (pectoralis major) covers the whole front area of the ribs, like a plaster. It runs over the collarbone, breastbone and ribs in several layers to the bones in the upper arm, and is responsible for the raising of the arms, amongst other things. The muscle is surrounded by the chest fascia (pectoral fascia) and connected to the abdominal fascia.

You need: Fascia ball, tennis ball
Come into an upright, comfortable seated position. In order to roll the left side of the chest muscle, place the fascia ball on the muscle with the right hand. Begin to roll the chest muscles in circular movements wherever it feels good to do so. Move from one side to the other underneath the collarbone. After approximately one minute, change to the other side. To roll the right side of the chest muscle, roll the fascia ball with the left hand. This ensures the part being rolled remains relaxed.

Note: Feel free to pause at tense areas and deepen your breathing. As you breathe in, the chest expands and the pressure in the area you are rolling increases. As you breathe out, the chest closes again and the pressure is reduced. Stay in this area for four to five breaths. Close your eyes in order to remain fully focused on the chest muscles and your breathing.

Benefits for your yoga practice
Rolling the chest area opens the front of your body at the level of your arms. You will become more open in the chest area and have increased arm mobility for backward and upward movements. Rolling before heart-opening exercises and back bends from the upper body helps to make the front of the upper body more supple.

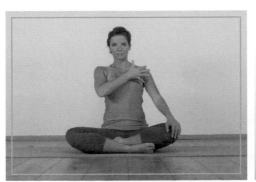
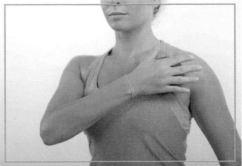

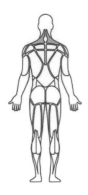

Neck

The neck area is very complex, and includes both surface and deep muscles. The muscles are layered on top of each other, and are all connected with a strong neck fascia. This area of fascia runs from the upper shoulder area over the whole head to the eyebrows.

You need: Fascia roller

Lie on your back in a comfortable position. Place the roller underneath your neck and rest your arms at the sides of your body. Slowly turn the head from one side to the other, as if drawing a semicircle in the air with the tip of your nose. Close your eyes and enjoy the relaxation.

Benefits for your yoga practice

Our neck is often put under a lot of stress. Even small changes in posture can mean that the neck muscles have to carry much more weight than they are designed for. Over the long term, this tires the muscles and they begin to stiffen. This results in tension in the neck. By working the muscles in the back of the neck, you can gently loosen some of this tension, and keep the muscles supple in the future. Rolling the neck is recommended as preparation for all poses, as it has a positive effect on our general well-being and awareness of the body.

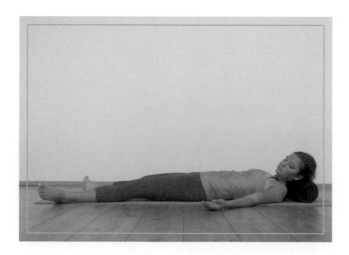

Which exercise is best when?

As a result of the increased circulation and loosened tensions, your movements will be more supple. You can make your practice easier by properly preparing your body. But, often, we don't have time to roll the whole body. The following table gives you some guidance. After an intensive, strong yoga session, it can also be a good idea to relax the muscles and fascia activated by the practice with targeted rolling.

Yoga practice	Preparation with the roller or ball
Downward-facing dog (page 54)	Soles of the feet, calves, hamstrings, buttocks, thoracic vertebrae, chest
Cobra, upward-facing dog (page 64)	Thighs, chest, thoracic vertebrae
Warrior (page 62)	Chest muscles, thighs
Standing forward fold (page 52)	Soles of the feet, calves, hamstrings, buttocks, lumbar vertebrae, thoracic vertebrae, neck
Triangle (page 76)	Inner thighs, buttocks, side body
Extended side angle (page 77)	Inner thighs, buttocks, side body
Revolved side angle (page 81)	Hip flexors, buttocks, lumbar vertebrae, thoracic vertebrae, chest
Focus	**Preparatory exercises**
Forward bends	Soles of the feet, Achilles tendon, hamstrings, buttocks, lower back, upper back, neck
Back bends	Shins, thighs, chest
Twists	Outer thighs, buttocks, side body, upper back
Side bends	Outer thighs, side body, lower back, upper back
Hip openers	Buttocks, outer thighs, inner thighs, lower back

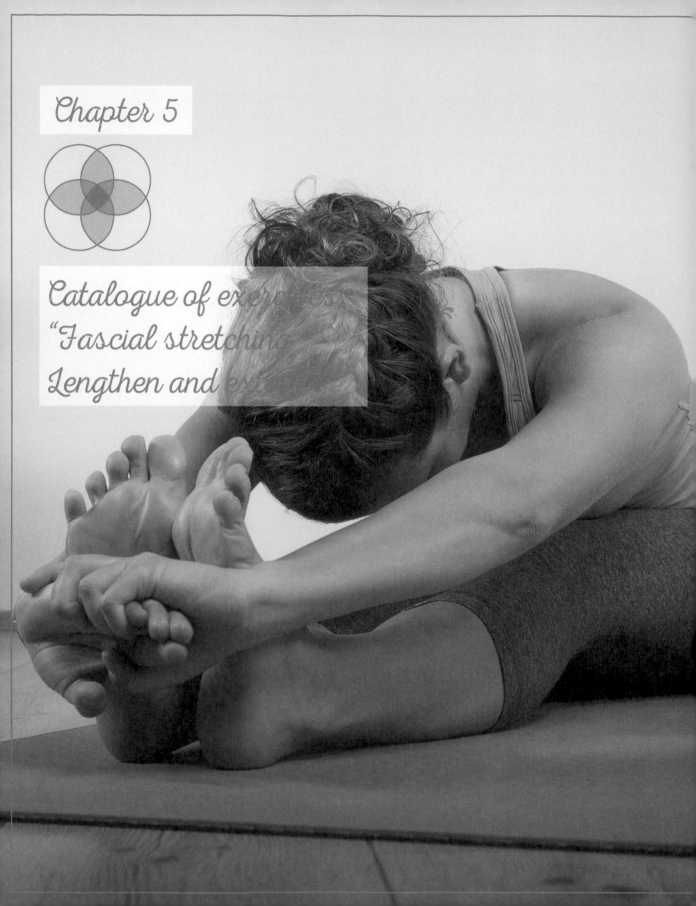

Chapter 5

Catalogue of exercises
"Fascial stretching"
Lengthen and ext

Is yoga fascial training? Definitely. Fascia is a very diverse, multifunctional tissue that needs a variety of movements to stimulate the different parts we have already learned about (collagen, elastin, connective tissue cells, ground substance, etc.). With static stretching alone, you will reach some of the fascia, but not all.

All stretching is not made equal

How does the traditional stretching we do in yoga differ from fascia yoga? Movement! Fascia loves movement. This guideline will also be put into practice in the following exercise section. We will be applying two basic techniques in order to make the yoga poses more stimulating.

» **Slow, fluid movements with many changes in direction**
Don't think of the poses as static positions that you move into for a few breaths and then move out of. Play with the pose! Stretch as far as you can, then extend in all directions. Change the direction of the stretch, with the idea of slowly melting further into the pose. Always think about two or three directions in which you want to extend.

Scientific background

The aim of this is to bring the alignment of the collagen fibres into a criss-crossed network – like the netting around vegetables in a supermarket. Stretching movements are necessary to align the collagen structures, as they stimulate the connective tissue cells to create collagen. The newly formed collagen fibres align themselves according to the forces exerted on them. This is why, in fascia yoga, we use multidirectional stretching.

» **Small bouncing movements**
Bring life and movement to your yoga poses. Move into the pose and then begin to make small, conscious bouncing movements. Slight rocking or bouncing gives the fascial tissue more stretchability and elasticity, like a spring. Begin gently with small movements, and avoid expansive swinging movements when you have stretched as far as possible.

Scientific background

For a long time, these bouncing, dynamic methods of stretching were rather demonised and rejected in sports science. But current research shows that these methods have a positive impact. In chapter 6, you will learn more about the memory capacity of fascia.

Whatever method you decide to use, the following concepts are typical of fascia yoga:

» **Include long fascial chains**
The exercises in this book are designed to work with the long fascial chains. You'll learn which ones those are in this chapter. In principle, the focus in fascia yoga is not on individual parts of the body or a single muscle group, but rather on including the whole body at all times. You train a network that is present throughout the whole body. From head to toe.

» **Three-dimensional thinking**
When moving through your yoga practice, think in at least two, or even better three, dimensions. Expand into the space and stretch your fascial network in all possible directions in order to bring length and openness back to the body.

Tip: Visualise this expansion when you move in your poses. Develop your own internal body compass. Using the example of the standing forward fold, this means that, moving with awareness, you slide your sitting bones further towards the ceiling and, at the same time, slide the crown of your head towards the floor. On a compass, this would be an expansion to the north and south. Stretching in two directions gives your body length, both in the upper body (lengthening the spine) and in the legs.

» Changing direction and position

Change the pose. In fascia yoga, we aren't looking for the perfect alignment. Each body, each person, and each fascial network is different. Make the pose perfect for you by trying new things and finding what feels good for you. Even tiny changes, such as the position of the hands or feet, can give the pose a completely different feeling.

» Being dynamic

In fascia yoga, we avoid the static holding of poses. You are constantly moving. These movements can be very small. The tiniest micro-movements, almost invisible to anyone watching make all the difference. This dynamism can also be provided by your breathing.

» Mixing methods

It's all about the mix! Try both variations of stretching given in this book – the flowing changes of direction and the small rocking movements. You may develop a clear preference for one or the other. Or maybe you'll prefer different methods for different poses. Be aware and develop a way of changing methods that is meaningful for you. Fascia yoga is playful, multifaceted and, above all, individual.

It is an invitation to try out new ways of moving. Make fascia yoga exercises a personal experience for you alone.

It is not a question of doing everything perfectly – what counts is how you experience the practice. Be creative!

Back fascial chain

The back fascial chain is an interconnected band running from under the toes up the back of the body to the back of the head, over the crown and to the eyebrows. It connects the soles of the feet, Achilles tendons, calf muscles, hamstrings, back extensors, neck and the plate of connective tissue that covers the skull.

The back fascial chain allows us to stand up straight, as it connects various points that are important for keeping the body upright. If you think about your body, you'll notice that many parts of the back fascial chain show a high level of fascial tension: the Achilles tendon, the muscles in the backs of your legs, and the long muscles in your back. Intense full-time demands are placed on these muscles and fascia as a result of the constant stresses of keeping us upright.

The back fascial chain can be split into two parts with different functions:

» Soles of the feet to the knee
» Knee to scalp

When the knees are straight, the back fascial chain works as a complete unit. This connection is lost when the knees are bent slightly. In yoga, this connection is very important. Bent knees give more mobility in the pelvic area, as the back fascial chain is not under stress. For this reason, I recommend bending the knees slightly when moving the spine. The pelvis is the initiator of the movement, regardless of the direction in which the spine is moving.

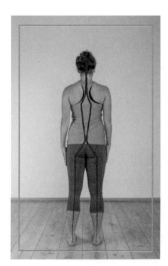

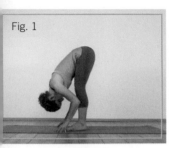

Fig. 1

Standing forward fold

» Stand upright and bend the knees a little.
» Tilt your pelvis forward slightly. Bend forwards from the hips until your fingertips or hands reach the mat. Keep length through the spine and relax your neck. Let your head, shoulders and arms hang. Surrender yourself to gravity.

Note: Bend your knees so that your fingertips or hands reach the mat.

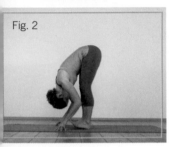

Fig. 2

Variation 1: Extending the back fascial chain by transfering your weight

» Transfer your weight to your heels so you can lift the toes and, if possible, the balls of your feet. Straighten your knees a little more to strengthen the stretch in the back of your legs. At the same time, roll your head with awareness. Enjoy the stretch along the whole back fascial chain – from the soles of your feet to your head. Make sure to keep your hands on the floor and your shoulders relaxed (fig. 2).
» Place your toes back on the mat and bend your knees generously. Give your back length by aligning yourself with a straight back. This takes the stretch out of the back chain (fig. 3).

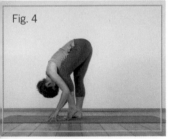

Fig. 3

Breathing: Connect your breathing with your movements. Exhale as you lift your toes, and inhale as you bend your knees with awareness.

Repeat this sequence for around ten breaths. With each breath you will become aware of your back softening.

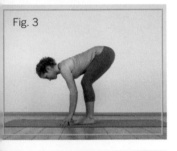

Fig. 4

Variation 2: Diagonal extension of the back fascial chain

» Change the position of your knees and hips. Bend and straighten the right and left knees alternately. Release your heels from the mat and let the movement extend to your hips. Include the buttocks, sliding the right and left side of the buttocks towards the ceiling in turn, and always with awareness (fig. 4).
» Let the movement grow. Include your whole body. Move the legs again, and move your arms forwards, alternating left and right. Extend diagonally. Try moving in all directions that are possible for you (fig. 5).

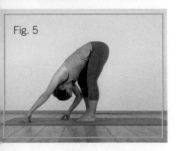

Fig. 5

These variations apply multidirectional tensile loads to the large back fascial chain.

Seated forward fold

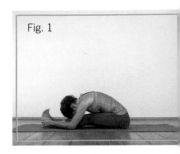

Fig. 1

» Sit on the mat with your legs out in front of you. Root your sitting bones into the mat and, at the same time, lengthen through your spine, so that you are sitting straight and upright. Move the insides of the feet together, slide the heels forwards and pull the toes back towards the upper body.

» From the pelvis, move the upper body forwards. Hold the outsides of your feet, your ankles or your shins. Keep as much length in the spine as possible. Move the breastbone and the pelvic bone away from each other. The shoulders and neck remain relaxed. The head hangs in order to include the top part of the back fascial chain in the stretch (fig. 1).

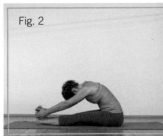

Fig. 2

Variation 1: Rounded back

» Clasp your hands to your feet, ankles or shins. You can use a towel to help if necessary. Roll it lengthways or diagonally into a strap, hold the ends and place it around the soles of your feet. Round your back with awareness. Slide your heels forwards and press the hollows of your knees into the mat. Feel how this lengthens the backs of your legs. Slide your spine and sitting bones backwards and hold yourself steady with your hands. This brings your whole back into the stretch. Breathe into your rounded back with awareness (fig. 2).

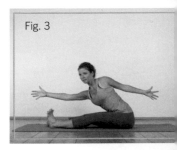

Fig. 3

In yoga, the traditional forward bend is generally taught with a straight back. This works the back extensors, which in turn puts pressure on the back muscles and stretches the spine. Try the rounded back variation as a "fascial" alternative. By curving the back, you take the muscular stress out of this area and move into the deeper fascial tissue.

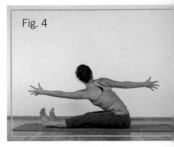

Fig. 4

Variation 2: Diagonal extension when sitting

» Gently slide the left and right feet forwards alternately. The movement comes from your hips. When you move the right hip forward, pull the left hip back with awareness, and vice versa. The legs remain straight and the upper body is folded forward. At the same time, move your arms forward alternately, in a diagonal direction. This includes the whole body in the stretch (figs 3 and 4).

» Vary the movement and connect the various directions in a flowing movement. Move your spine in all directions possible for you. Be creative and find what feels good (fig. 5).

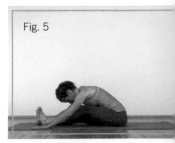

Fig. 5

Downward-facing dog

» Come into tabletop position and align yourself here (see page 26).
» On an exhalation, move your buttocks upwards towards the ceiling. At first, keep your knees slightly bent. This makes the pelvis more mobile. You can bring more length to your spine by tilting your pelvis backwards. Stretch your back. Slide your breastbone backwards towards your knees. Centre your arms. It may help you to imagine that you have an orange in each armpit, and want to press it. Move your shoulders away from your ears – this provides a powerful level of stability.
» Slowly and gently, stretch your knees backwards. Push your heels towards the back edge of the mat. Press upwards with strength, as if you were pushing the mat forwards and away. As seen from the side, your body forms an upside-down V shape (fig. 1).

Tip: You can keep your legs bent! It's always more important to keep your back long and stretched than to straighten your legs. If a lack of mobility in your shoulders makes it difficult to bring your arms into a diagonal line, bend your knees a little more (fig. 2).

Variation 1: Big dog

» Slide further upwards from downward dog. To do this, come onto your toes and lift your heels up as far as possible. Your buttocks move straight up. Move the upper and lower body closer together, without changing the position of your hands and feet on the mat (fig. 3).
» Return your heels to the mat and slide a little further into the mat with awareness. If you can, lift your toes off the mat (fig. 4).

Breathing: Let both movements become a flow. As you inhale, move higher, and as you exhale, ground your body again.

Variation 2: Lolling dog
This variation turns downward-facing dog into a playground for moving your whole body.

» First, bring movement to your feet and knees by slowly walking on the spot and bending and stretching each knee alternately. You'll feel the stretch in the backs of your legs change.
» Make your movements bigger and include the hips, moving them in circles or from side to side. This changes the level of tension in the large back fascia (fig. 5).

» Let the movement shift to your spine and play with the range of motion your spine offers: bend, stretch, rotate and move side to side. Move the spine in waves and snakelike patterns while in downward-facing dog. You'll notice that your shoulders are also included in the movement (fig. 6).

Lolling dog is a wonderful fascia stretch. Guide your movements to individual joints (feet, knees, hips, spine, shoulders) one at a time, developing your awareness of your range of motion. Finally, connect all your joints, bending and stretching your whole body in a flowing movement. Find what feels best for you – your "feel-good dog".

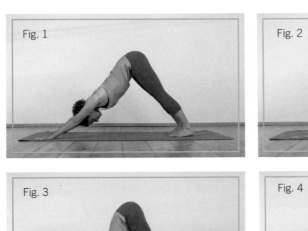

Fig. 1

Fig. 2

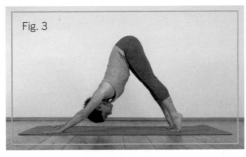

Fig. 3

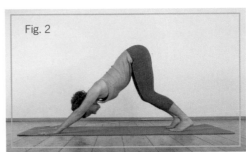

Fig. 4

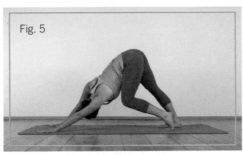

Fig. 5

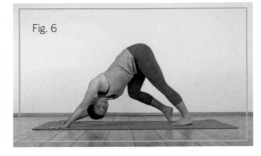

Fig. 6

Plow

» Begin lying on your back, and lay your arms straight out next to the body. Bend your knees and lift your legs off the floor. Lift your hips too. Support your pelvis from underneath by placing your hands either side of your spine (fig. 1).
» Move your knees further backwards over your head and straighten your legs until your toes touch the floor. If you can, place your arms flat on the floor. In this position, your back can be more rounded. Your weight rests on your shoulders, not on your neck (fig. 2).

Tip: If you can't reach the floor with your feet, you can practise plow using a wall. Support yourself with your feet where you can reach the wall easily (fig. 3).

Only stay in the pose for as long as it is comfortable. If you feel pressure in your head or your cervical spine, slowly come out of the pose. The wall variation may be a good idea if this is the case.

Breathing: Use your breathing to make small, subtle movements that create more length. The movements will be barely visible to anyone watching, but you will certainly feel them! As you breathe in, move your heels and buttocks away from each other. Slide your heels further backwards and down, and the buttocks forwards and upwards. Think in both directions, and extend as far as you can. Release with your exhalation (fig. 4).

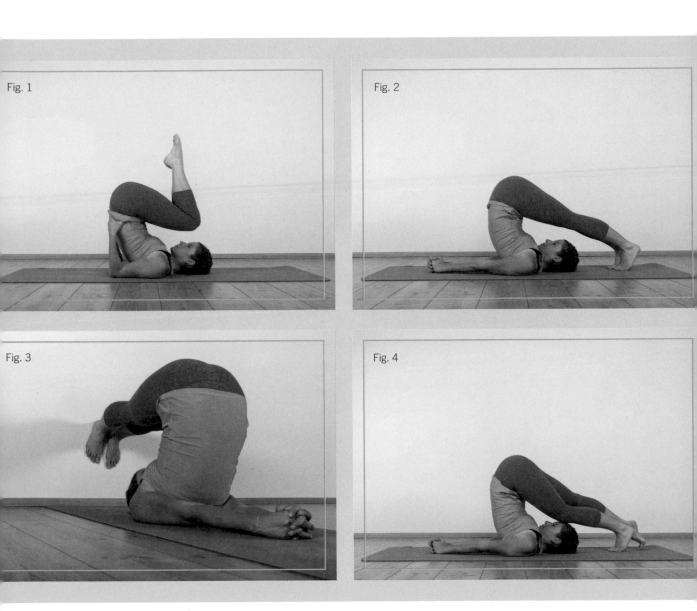

Fig. 1

Fig. 2

Fig. 3

Fig. 4

Half pyramid

» Begin in high lunge (page 26). Place your back knee on the mat. From there, slide backwards with your buttocks, while slowly stretching your front leg. Pull the toes of your front leg towards your shin. Expand and lengthen your back. Tilt your pelvis forwards slightly in order to lengthen your lower back. Move your heart centre forwards and your buttocks backwards. Move in both directions with awareness. Make sure that both hipbones remain aligned at the same height (fig. 1).

» Move your upper body over your outstretched leg with soft, small, wavelike movements.

Tip: If your back is rounded, place your hands under your shoulders and move onto your fingertips. This helps the upper body to be more aligned and makes it easier for you to stretch your back.

Variation: Exploring the pyramid

» Go on a voyage of discovery! Change the position of your hands. Bring both hands to one side of your leg, or move one hand further forward. Stretch lengthways and diagonally. Include your arms, shoulders, spine and hips. Think in three dimensions (figs 2 and 3).

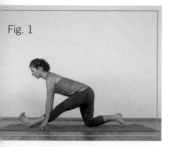
Fig. 1

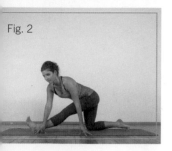
Fig. 2

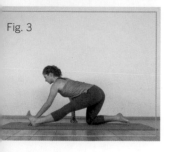
Fig. 3

Relaxation for the back fascial chain - child's pose

» From tabletop position (see page 26), slowly slide your buttocks backwards onto your heels. Lay your forehead on the mat and your arms to the sides of your body. Let your shoulders sink gently and easily downwards (fig. 1).

If you can't easily reach your heels with your buttocks, it may be helpful to place a cushion or a blanket between your buttocks and your heels. If placing your forehead on the mat is not comfortable for you, bend your arms and lay your forehead on your hands.

Tip: Move the knees further apart and allow your upper body to sink even lower between your legs. This opens the hips further and allows the body to expand.

Variation: Moving child

» In child's pose, stretch your arms out in front of you. This lengthens your spine and expands the shoulders.
» As you inhale, start to move your upper body in wavelike patterns. Round your back and roll with your head. As you exhale, slide back again onto your heels, lengthening the spine again (fig. 2).
» Vary the position of the arms. Stretch your arms to the right or left, and repeat the movement as described (fig. 3).

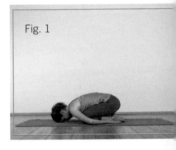

Fig. 1

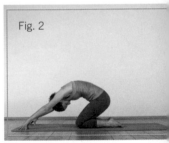

Fig. 2

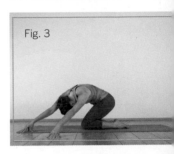

Fig. 3

Cat

» Come into tabletop position (page 26). Begin to round the spine from the pelvis. To do this, tilt your pelvis backwards and tuck your tailbone forwards and under. Your chin moves towards your breastbone. Gently draw your belly button inwards and actively press your mat away with your hands. Your shoulder blades will be stretched and your neck lengthened. Make sure your shoulders are drawn away from your ears and that they stay over your wrists (fig. 1).

Variation: Wild cat

» Make your cat lively and wild. Slide more to the side and upwards, or press your thoracic spine upwards with awareness. Try it out, and play with your spine (figs 2 and 3).

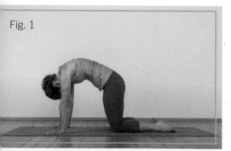

Fig. 1

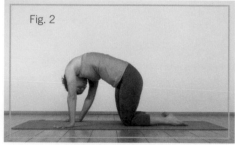

Fig. 2

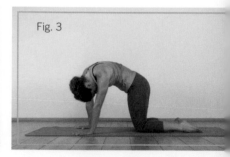

Fig. 3

Front fascial chain

The front fascial chain, which also comprises two parts, connects the whole front of the body from the tops of the feet to the sides of the skull. The lower part runs from the toes to the pelvis, and connects the toe extensors, shins, kneecaps and patellar tendons as well as the four-headed thigh muscle. This part ends at the front edge of the large triangular pelvic bone. The upper part runs from the pelvis to the head and connects the bump of the pubic bone, the abdominal fascia (all four areas of the abdominal muscles), the ribs, breastbone, the muscles that flex the neck and the skull.

The front fascial chain can be seen as the counterpart to the back fascial chain. According to the fascia principle that "everything is connected to everything else", both chains are connected through the outer tissue layers of the toes. While the back fascial chain is primarily responsible for our posture, the muscles in the front fascial chain are always ready to protect the soft, sensitive parts of the body. Due to anxiety and protective reflexes, our front fascial chain tends to shorten in order to protect the vulnerable vital organs (for example the lungs and the heart). In fascia yoga, our goal is to open this front chain.

If the hips are stretched, the front fascial chain works as a continuous line of tension. When the hips move, this line is broken. This explains why, for example, in cow pose (see page 69), only part of the front chain is reached, not the whole chain, as the stress is taken out of the lower part by the movement of the hips.

Back bends stretch the front fascial chain and promote a certain level of mobility in the spine and pelvis. Start with the first exercises (warrior, cobra and bridge pose). If these feel good, gradually begin the other, more advanced exercises.

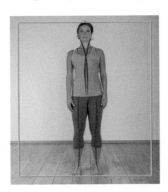

Warrior

Warrior is an asymmetrical standing back bend. In the basic position, the upper part of the front fascial chain is stretched. The stretch is then extended down from the hip on one side, via the hip flexor to the knee of the straight leg.

» Begin in high lunge (page 26). Stabilise your legs with awareness by stretching the back leg, activating the thigh muscle and sliding the heel upwards.
» Lift your upper body up and forwards until the shoulders are aligned over the hips. Move your arms from your sides upwards next to the ears. Maintain tension in your legs (back leg actively stretched, front knee over the ankle joint). Make sure that both hip bones are facing forwards. Move the pelvic bone up and forwards. Activate your abdominal muscles. Lift your heart centre forwards and upwards, sliding the shoulders back and down. This lengthens the upper body (fig. 1).

Tip: Always align yourself from your feet upwards. The stronger and more stable your legs and pelvis, the more ease and freedom you will have in the upper body. This will make the alignment of the spine, shoulders and arms much easier.

In traditional yoga, warrior is usually practised with the back heel down on the mat. In fascia yoga we use a variation with a lifted heel, as this offers the following benefits:

» Optimal tension in the front fascial chain (so the spiral fascial chain is not involved)
» Slight forward alignment of the hips, as the back hip is more mobile
» Correct alignment of the knee axis, even with less mobile hips.

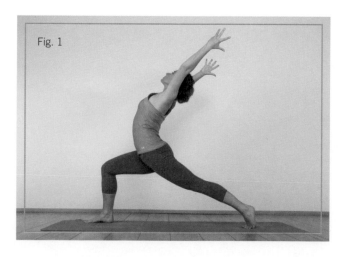

Fig. 1

Fascia tip: Gentle bouncing with the upper body
Move your arms a little further backwards with gentle pulsing movements. Open your shoulders and chest. Include the whole body in your bouncing. At the same time, keep your abdominal muscles active, so that your trunk and legs remain stable (fig. 2).

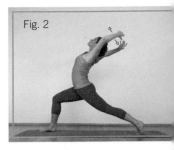

Fig. 2

Gentle bouncing gradually opens the front body, so that you feel taller and softer. Begin with very small movements, becoming bigger as you gain more experience in your practice.

Variation: Fighting warrior

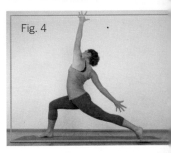

Fig. 3

» Come into a stable warrior pose and start to move your upper body freely. Stretch in various directions. Your spine should experience all possible directions of movement. Rotate, lean to each side, curve and stretch. Or connect the different options together. Bring the stretch into your fingertips and picture how you are stretching your fascial chain in all possible directions (figs 3–5).

Breathing: As you inhale, expand and stretch in all directions. As you exhale, come back to centre, ready to stretch in another direction on your next inhalation.

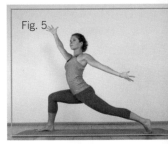

Fig. 4

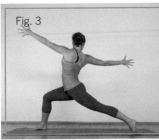

Fig. 5

Cobra

» Lie on your stomach and place your hands either side of your body, under your shoulders. Keep your elbows close to the body.
» Roll your shoulders back and down with awareness. Press yourself upwards gently, using your arms to lift the upper body. Move your breastbone upwards and forwards. It should feel as if you are pushing your mat back away from you. This creates length in the upper body and reduces the pressure on the lower back. Your feet should be hip width apart at most, and your buttocks relaxed (fig. 1).

If you feel pressure in your lower back, keep your upper body closer to the ground. In cobra, the idea is not to come as high as possible. Cobra is a heart-opening pose, with your focus placed on the thoracic spine. The breastbone moves forwards, and the shoulders sink down the back. This pose counteracts the natural curvature of the spine (kyphotic curve).

Fascia tip: Bend a leg as you lift
As you inhale, lift one leg to extend the tension into the front fascial chain of the bent leg. As you exhale, return the upper body and the leg to the mat. Repeat the variation of the exercise on the other side (fig. 2).

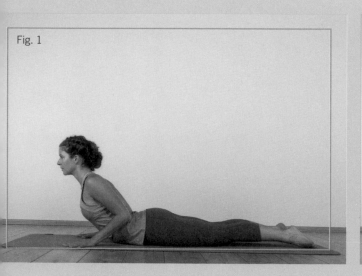

Fig. 1

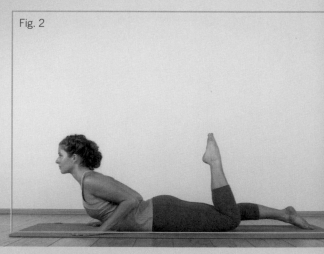

Fig. 2

Variation 1: Curious cobra

» Release your hands from the mat and move your arms and upper body freely.
  Move one arm forwards and the other backwards, both arms forwards or both arms
  backwards. Be curious and move your head too, looking over your left and right
  shoulders in turn (fig. 3).
» Lift one or both legs as you lift your upper body, to bring the whole body into the
  stretch. Imagine your body getting longer and longer as you push your toes away
  (fig. 4).

Variation 2: Upward-facing dog
Upward-facing dog is a more intense variation for stretching the front fascial chain. It is
more suited to experienced yogis.

» Begin in the same starting position as for cobra. With this variation, push yourself
  higher by straightening your arms further. Activate your leg muscles and rotate the
  upper legs inwards slightly in order to widen the lower back. Straighten your arms
  as far as is comfortable for your back. The shoulder blades move down and back
  towards the pelvis. The waist is long and the heart centre lifted forward.
» Lift your knees from the mat, so that only your palms and the tops of your feet are
  touching the mat. The shoulders should be aligned above the wrists. Keep length
  in the sacral area and lower back. Here, it is primarily the upper back that is being
  involved in the back bend (fig. 5).

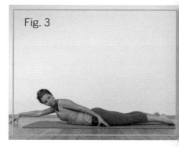

Fig. 3

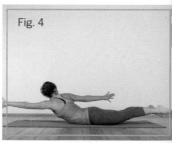

Fig. 4

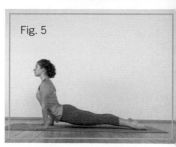

Fig. 5

Bridge

» Lie on your back and place your feet near your buttocks. The arms rest at the sides of the body. Nestle the lower back firmly into the mat and slowly, starting with the tailbone, roll the spine upwards. The muscles in the buttocks are active and push the hip bones up further. The thighs remain parallel (fig. 1).

Tip: When your pelvis is lifted, pull your shoulders closer together under your upper body and interlock your hands under your body. Push the breastbone up further, allowing you to open the upper body even more.

Variation 1: Pelvic swing

» Come into bridge pose and place your arms about shoulder width from your body. Start moving the pelvis from side to side. Keep the buttocks high. Explore other possible movements, such as rocking the knees back and forth or making circling movements (figs 2 and 3).

Tip: Close your eyes to bring your senses inward. Concentrate all your awareness on your pelvis and its range of motion. Become aware of the openness and mobility of the front fascial chain.

Variation 2: Wheel
This heart-opening back bend requires a high level of strength and mobility in the shoulders. It is more suited to experienced yogis.

» Lie on your back and place your feet near your buttocks. Bend your arms and place the palms on the mat near your ears. The fingertips face slightly outwards. The elbows are as close together as possible.
» Slowly lift your pelvis and press upwards strongly through your hands and feet. Use the strength in your legs to push the upper body further backwards. The breastbone floats upwards and the shoulders are open. The goal is to create an elliptical shape with your body, rather than a semi-circle. This puts less pressure on the lower back and the main back bend is focused in the upper body (fig. 4).

Tip: The distance between your hands and feet determines how strong the pose is. Placing the feet further away from the hands reduces the stress on the spine. I recommend a larger distance.

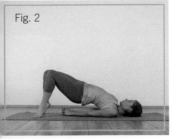
Fig. 1

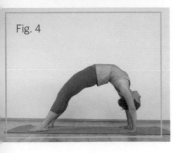
Fig. 2

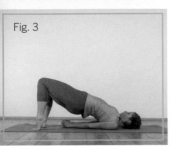
Fig. 3

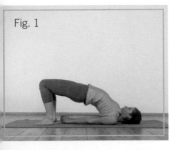
Fig. 4

Camel

» Begin in kneeling pose (page 25). Lift the buttocks, bringing the knees, pelvis and shoulders into a single line. Place your hands on your hips. Activate your abdominal muscles to stabilise your lower back. Roll your shoulders back and pull the elbows closer to the body.

» Now lean back from your knees. The upper body and thighs remain almost in line. The hips remain stretched and the lower back is long (fig. 5).

» Hold your heels to the left and right. The thumbs face inwards, and the fingers outwards. Open the shoulders as wide as possible. Let the breastbone lift to the ceiling (fig. 6).

Variation: One-armed camel

» Move into camel pose. Release your right arm from your heel and bring it forwards and upwards. Pull the arm backwards as far as possible, so that it continues the alignment of the body. This movement of the arm extends the stretch in the front fascial chain (fig. 7).

» Before moving to the other side, take a break and lower your buttocks to the mat. Then repeat with the left arm.

Fascia tip: Rocking arm
Gently rocking the outstretched arm sends small pulsing movements into the front fascial chain.

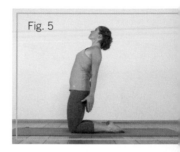
Fig. 5

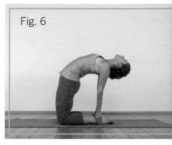
Fig. 6

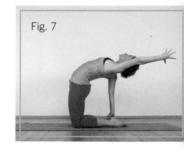
Fig. 7

Bow

» Lie on your stomach and bend both legs. Take hold of the outsides of your feet or your ankles with your hands. The knees and feet are hip width apart. Push the lower legs backwards and slowly lift the upper body. Imagine that your legs are trying to straighten, but your hands are stopping them. Push your heart centre forward. Keep length in the waist. Draw your belly button towards your spine in order to avoid pressing the abdomen into the mat.

» Lift your thighs. Activate the legs, allowing your upper body to remain relaxed. Just like in cobra, the goal is not to be as upright as possible, but rather to open the whole front body equally (fig. 1).

Fascia tip: Vary your grip
Hold the insides of the feet with both hands and observe how this changes the openness of the upper body (fig. 2). Hold your toes in order to target the whole front fascial chain (fig. 3).

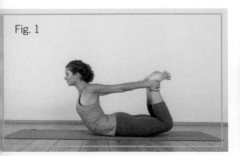
Fig. 1

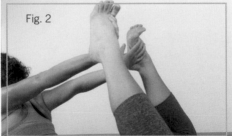
Fig. 2

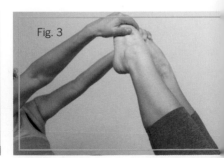
Fig. 3

Relaxation for the front fascial chain - cow

» Begin in tabletop position (page 26). Tilt your pelvis forward. The sitting bones move up and back. Your spine slides vertebra by vertebra into a gentle back bend. If it is comfortable for you, allow the front body to hang down. Push your breastbone forward. Your gaze is also directed forwards. Your spine forms a long, soft arc from the tailbone to the back of your head (fig. 1).

Fascia tip: Alternating cat–cow
Cat (see page 60) and cow can be combined to create a wonderful stretch for both the front and back fascial chains. Move into cat as you exhale and into cow as you inhale (fig. 2).

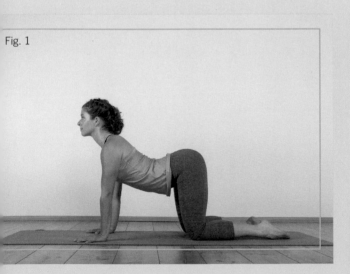

Fig. 1

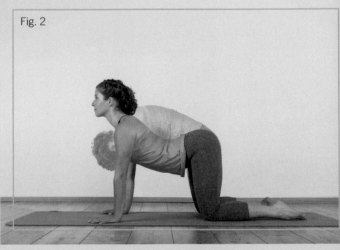

Fig. 2

Fish using a meditation cushion

» Sit on the mat with your legs out in front of you. Place a meditation cushion approximately 30 cm behind you on the mat and roll backwards onto the cushion. The cushion should be under your thoracic spine area. Spread your arms out to the sides and surrender to the stretch (fig. 1). Let yourself fall completely. Let go!

Tip: The closer the cushion is to your buttocks, the more intensely you'll feel the opening and stretching into the spine area. If the cushion is further from your buttocks, your chest will be opened less.

Fascia tip: Move the arms upwards for more length
Stretch your arms upwards, with the palms facing up (fig. 2). This provides an optimal stretch for the front fascial chain and allows you to lengthen further. Having your arms to the sides creates width and space. Vary your position.

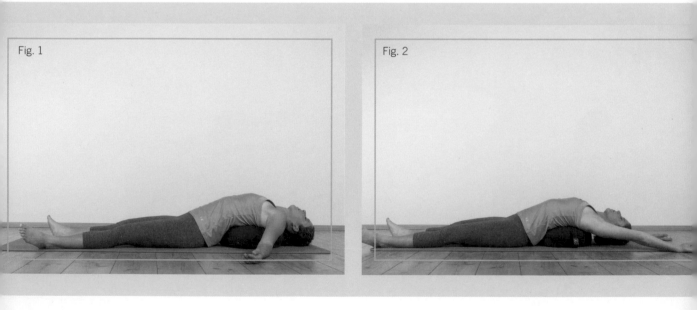

Fig. 1

Fig. 2

Side fascial chains

The side fascial chains, also called lateral lines, bracket the body from both sides like a container. This is why we cannot talk about one fascial chain – there are two of them: one fascia band on each side, right and left, pulling upwards. They start in the middle of the outside of the foot and run over the outside of the ankle, the leg and upwards. They cover the lateral ribs in a widespread wickerwork pattern and then pass under the shoulders and up to the sides of the skull at ear level.

The side fascial chains act as a connection between the front and back fascial chains. They ensure the proper balance and exchange between both sides. They fix the trunk and legs, while the arms can move freely. Due to their role in stabilising the pelvis and trunk, and the interconnections in the rib area, they can also be used as "brakes" when rotating the trunk. In terms of function, the side fascial chains are involved in all side bends of the trunk and splaying of the legs. If they are stretched on one side, they contract on the other.

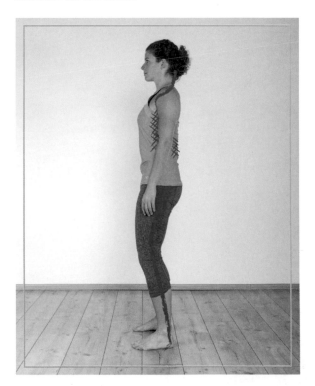

Standing crescent

» Stand in an upright position and root your feet into the mat (see page 23). As you exhale, lift your arms straight up from your sides. The palms face each other. Bring length to the spine. The shoulders remain low and the neck is relaxed.
» Lean the whole upper body to the right from the hips. Push the fingertips of your left hand further upwards and to the right. Try to extend upwards rather than lean to the side. The left side body is lengthened, but the right side is not shorter (fig. 1). Root your left foot into the mat with awareness so that you can stretch the body in two directions.
» Repeat this exercise on the other side (fig. 2).

Variation: Changing moon

» On an inhalation, lift your arms (mountain pose, see page 94).
» As you exhale, lean from the hips to the right side. Bring length to the left side body.
» As you inhale, come back to mountain pose and align yourself.
» As you exhale, lean from the hips to the left side. Now bring length to the right side body (fig. 2).

Fascia tip: Change the alignment of your hands
Vary the position of the hands. Rotate your palms inwards and outwards in order to vary the tensile load on the side fascial chains. Include your shoulders in the movement (fig. 2).

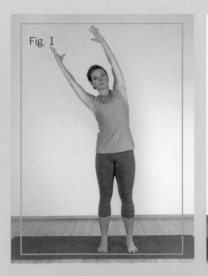
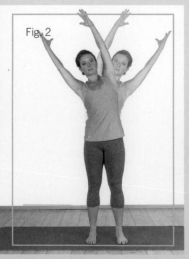

Fig. 1

Fig. 2

Shoelace with side bend

» Sit upright with your legs out straight in front of you. Bend your right leg and lay it over the left leg. The outer edge or top of the foot touches the floor near the left buttock (fig. 1).

» Bend the left leg. Move the left heel closer to the right buttock. If it is comfortable for you, move the knees one on top of the other (fig. 2).

» Lift the left arm and stretch upwards from the side body. With your upper body, come into a side bend to the right. Support yourself by resting your right hand on the floor. Take care to keep your shoulders relaxed on both sides, for both the straight and supporting arms (fig. 3).

Tip: Raise your sitting position if you find that sitting upright in this position is difficult, or if you feel your pelvis tilting to one side. You'll find it easier to align your pelvis on a meditation cushion or blanket.

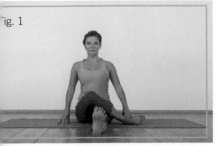

Fig. 1

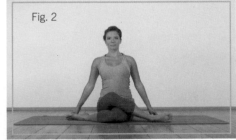

Fig. 2

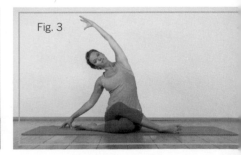

Fig. 3

Side arch

» Come into kneeling pose (page 25). Lift the left arm straight up from the side. Lean to the right from the upper body. Support yourself with your right arm to the side. Pull both shoulders away from your ears. Repeat this exercise on the other side (fig. 1).

Fascia tip: Increasing the arch with support
Side arch is a wonderful way to reach the upper side fascial chains. The lower part is left out owing to the seated position. Use a meditation cushion, yoga block or pile of books to help grow your arch. By lifting your buttocks, you can spread the arch further (fig. 2).

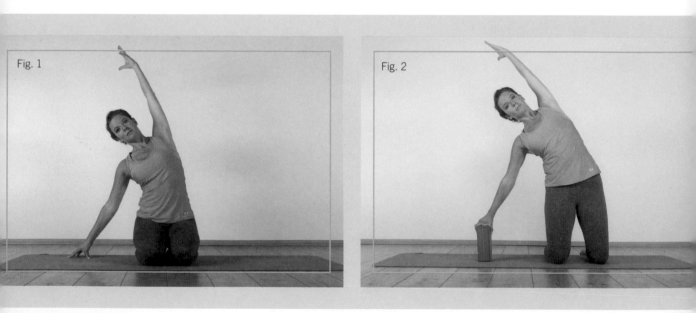

Fig. 1

Fig. 2

Gate pose

» Move from side arch (see page 74) to gate pose by stretching your left leg out to the side. Press the outer edge of the foot firmly into the floor, and at the same time lengthen through the left arm. Think in both directions to fully stretch your side fascial chain (fig. 1).
» Repeat this exercise on the other side (fig. 2).

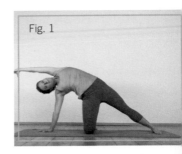

Fig. 1

Fascia tip: Connect your breathing with the movement
As you inhale, stretch to the right, and come back as you exhale. With your next inhalation, stretch to the left. Repeat this gentle opening swinging movement for eight to ten breaths. With each breath, bring a little more length to the side body. You will become soft and supple.

Variation: "Up and down" gate

» As you inhale, move to the right in gate pose. Stretch your body from the outer edge of your left foot to your left fingertips (fig. 3).
» With an exhalation, place your buttocks to the right, next to your right ankle, and place your left hand on the outside of your outstretched left leg. Lift your right arm and stretch it over to the left. Lean your upper body to the side in order to lengthen through the right side body (fig. 4).
» Repeat the alternating stretching, lifting and sitting for around ten breaths and then move to the other side.

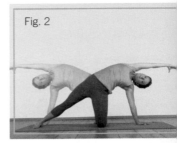

Fig. 2

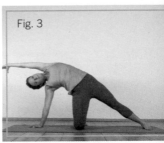

Fig. 3

Vary the alignment of your hands and shoulders. Point the thumb to the ceiling, or turn your palms upwards. Open your chest by pulling your shoulders back, or close it by leaning forwards. Be playful and creative in these flowing movements – up and down, stretching and relaxing in your own way. You will notice that stretching in various directions significantly increases your mobility in gate pose.

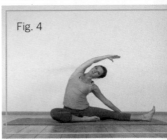

Fig. 4

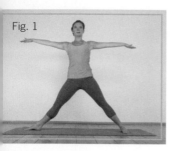

Fig. 1

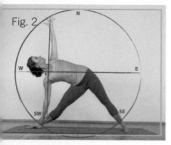

Fig. 2

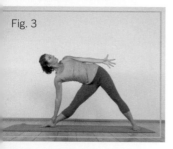

Fig. 3

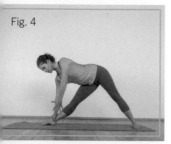

Fig. 4

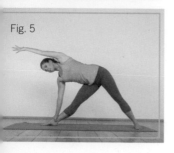

Fig. 5

Triangle

» Stand on the mat with the feet apart. The left foot is towards the front edge of the mat, and the right foot towards the back. The feet are approximately leg length apart and parallel. Turn the left foot 90° so that the toes are pointing forward. Activate your thigh muscles. Stretch the arms to the sides, at shoulder height. The backs of the hands face upwards (fig. 1).

» Move the whole upper body towards the right thigh from the hips. Keeping length in the spine, lean the upper body downwards. Place your right hand on your shin or ankle, or on the floor. Move the left arm straight up so that both arms are in line and the shoulders are aligned vertically. Look towards your left fingertips. Open your front body. Bring length to both sides of the upper body. If you notice that you are buckling at the waist and losing length in the spine, move your outstretched hand upwards (fig. 2).

» Repeat the exercise on the other side.

Fascia tip: Stretching in all directions
Imagine stretching your body in all directions of the compass (fig. 2):

» The top arm pulls upwards to the north, and the lower arm sinks down to the south. This expands the heart centre and brings ease to the arms.

» As you look at this photograph, the crown of your head points to the left – figuratively to the east. And the buttocks pull to the right, or the west. This stretching brings length to the spine and keeps the waist stable.

» The legs stabilise and form a strong foundation for a mobile spine.

Variation: Circling triangle

» Move the arm stretched upwards in a large circle, from back to front and then upwards again. Imagine you are drawing a large circle in the air with your fingertips. Keep your legs and hips stable and fixed. Keep the spine long. With awareness, move your shoulders and upper body with the circling arm. You will be able to feel the pull on the side fascial chain change in the waist and rib areas (figs 3–5).

» Repeat this exercise on the other side.

Extended side angle

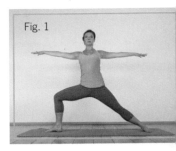

Fig. 1

» Stand on the mat with the feet apart. The right foot is towards the front edge of the mat, and the left foot towards the back. The feet are approximately leg length apart and parallel. Turn the left foot 90° so that the toes are pointing forward. Bend the front leg so that the knee is aligned over the heel. You can check that you are in the right position by looking to see if your big toe is still visible. The trunk is aligned over the pelvis, and the shoulders aligned directly above the hips.

» Activate the muscles in your buttocks and gently pull the tailbone up and forwards. Stretch the arms to the sides, at shoulder height. The backs of the hands face upwards. The shoulders remain relaxed (fig. 1).

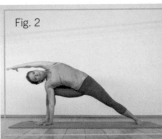

Fig. 2

» Lean your upper body to the right and place your right hand on the inside of your right foot. Bring your left arm straight over your head, so that if forms a line with your outstretched left leg. Open your heart centre upwards. Push the outer edge of your left foot firmly into the mat and, at the same time, lengthen your left arm. You will feel the right side body becoming longer and longer (fig. 2).

» Repeat the exercise on the other side.

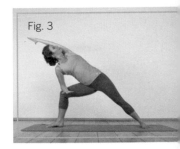

Fig. 3

Tip: You may not be able to reach the floor with your hand at first. If you feel your upper body sinking forward, support yourself with your forearm on the thigh. Make sure to pull your shoulders away from the ears (fig. 3).

Closely interwoven

As you'll have already noticed, many exercises can't be fully assigned to one fascial chain. Some poses are so complex that they include twists, forward bends, back bends and side bends, and therefore provide a mixture of different possible movements.

Triangle and extended side angle are a good demonstration of this. Carrying out both poses correctly is very much dependent on the mobility of the side fascial chain. This determines how far the upper body can be moved away from the hips. But the spiral fascial chain is just as important in both of these poses, as this is stretched to open the upper body upwards towards the ceiling. Both poses are well suited to maintaining balance between these two chains.

Relaxation for the side fascial chains – sideways child's pose

» Come into tabletop position (page 26). Move both hands 45° to the left on the mat (fig. 1).
» With your right arm, stretch further forwards and to the right. Walk your fingertips further forwards. At the same time, bend your left arm and lay your forehead on your forearm or on the back of your hand. The buttocks remain aligned over the knees. Your right shoulder sinks down, and the buttocks slide backwards (fig. 2). This creates space and length in your left side body.

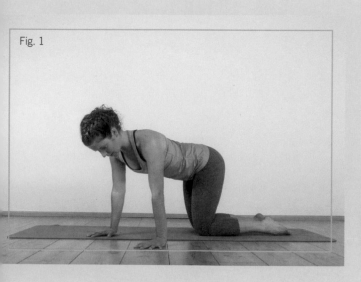

Fig. 1

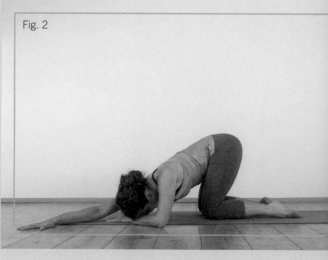

Fig. 2

Lying crescent

» Lie on your back with arms and legs spread wide, as if you wanted to make a big X shape with your body (fig. 1).
» Move your right foot to the left side. Bring your right arm to the left side too. Both arms and legs stay in contact with the floor. Your trunk and shoulders also remain on the floor. This provides the maximum stretch in your right side body. As seen from above, the X shape has now become a crescent moon (fig. 2).
» Repeat this exercise on the other side. First return to the X shape and stretch generously.

Tip: Close your eyes and breathe into the side of the body you are stretching with awareness. Lengthen along the whole side body. As you exhale, sink further and further into the mat with your whole body. As you exhale, release any tensions you feel into the mat.

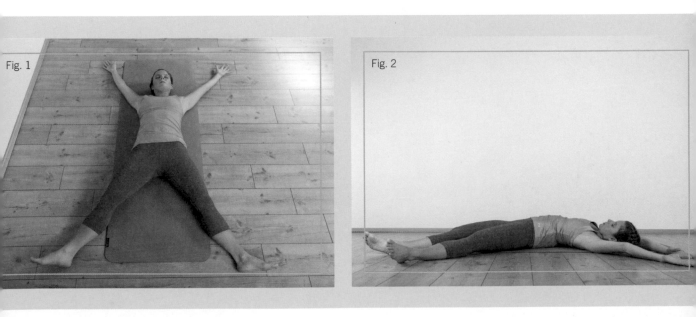

Fig. 1

Fig. 2

Spiral fascial chains

As with the side fascial chains, we also talk about the spiral fascial chains in the plural – there are two in our body. Both spiral chains run through our whole body, like a double helix. They run from the skull to the opposite shoulder and rib region, and along the oblique abdominal muscles back to the centre. They cross at the level of the belly button, leading to the hip on the same side of the body as they started at the skull. From the hips, they run down the front and side of the upper and lower leg to the inner arch of the foot and under the foot to the outside of the arch. The chain then runs back up the inner back of the leg, leading into the long back extensor fascia at the sitting bones. From there, they continue back up to the skull.

If the spiral fascial chains malfunction, for example in the form of tension, this can also have a negative effect on the other chains. Bad posture, such as pelvic misalignment, a head that tilts too far forward, hollow back and knees that are out of position, can stem from the spiral chains. This is why you should pay careful attention to your spiral fascial chains.

Twists and movements are particularly good at reaching the spiral fascial chains. Twists like the sitting half spinal twist (see page 87) or revolved side angle (see page 81) are well suited to stretching the upper part of the spiral chain, while the other side contracts. Pigeon (see page 85) is an excellent way to reach the lower part of the spiral chain.

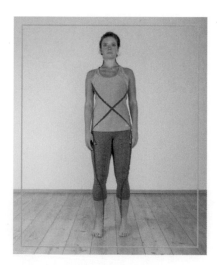

Revolved side angle

» Come into high lunge (page 26). Begin with the left foot to the front and the right foot back. Place your right hand to the inside of your left foot. Twist your upper body to the left and stretch your left arm upwards.
» Both arms form a straight vertical line. Open your left shoulder back, so that both shoulders are vertically aligned. Bring length into your spine to make the twist easier. Direct your gaze upwards past the fingertips of your left hand. This brings the whole spine, including the cervical spine, into the stretch (fig. 1). If the neck becomes tense, direct your gaze downwards towards your right hand.
» Repeat the exercise on the other side.

Tip: The closer your hand is to the inside of your foot, the more unstable the pose. The further away your hand, the more stable you will be.

Variation 1: Opening further in revolved side angle

» As you inhale, lower your back (right) knee to the mat. At the same time, extend further backwards with your left arm and twist further to the left. With the increased twist, your upper body no longer faces the side, but upwards. Ground your pelvis. The right hip bone moves further downwards, and the left hip bone upwards (fig. 2).
» As you exhale, return to the starting revolved side angle. The right knee is straightened and lifted from the mat. Repeat the intense opening and twisting for seven to ten breaths, then change to the other side.

Fascia tip: Hold, bounce and enjoy
You'll notice that as you breathe, you become softer and more mobile in the core and hip areas. Hold the fully open position for approximately five breaths and enjoy the space and openness in your whole body. With slight bouncing movements of the left arm, you can increase the opening of the shoulders and front body. As your whole body is interconnected, you'll feel these small pulsing movements down to your hips and legs. Try it out!

Variation 2: Circling angle

» Move your left arm back then down in a circle. Let your arm continue to circle past the front body upwards and then back to the starting position.
» Increase the size of your movements. You may like to bend your arm, or only circle your shoulder. Vary what you do and see what changes (figs 3–5).

Tip: The more stable your legs, the bigger and more creative you can be with your upper body. Your spine, shoulders and arms have more freedom to move and you can try more variations.

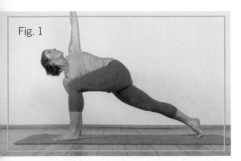

Fig. 1

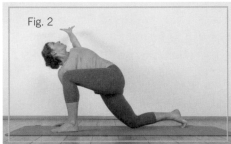

Fig. 2

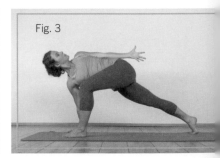

Fig. 3

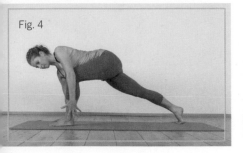

Fig. 4

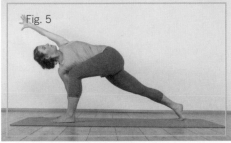

Fig. 5

Three-legged dog with twist

» Come into downward-facing dog (page 54). Lift your right foot from the floor and raise your leg, keeping it straight. The right hip bone rises further in order to open the hip upwards to the right. The shoulders remain level. Create as much length as possible (fig. 1).
» Keep the hips stable in this position. Activate your abdominal muscles, bend your right leg and pull the heel towards your buttocks. The right knee points upwards, and the right heel moves towards the left shoulder (fig. 2).
» Repeat the exercise on the other side.

Fascia tip: Pulsing heel
Gently pulse the heel of the bent leg in order to send small pulsing movements through the spiral fascial chains. Keep your abdominal muscles active.

Variation: Two-legged dog

» See this pose as a playful challenge. Come into three-legged dog with your right leg raised and bend your knee. Look under your left arm to see if your right heel is visible. If so, lift your left hand from the mat and take hold of your right foot (fig. 3).
» Be curious and playful! Even if you can't take hold of your foot, you will encourage balance in your body and stability in the spiral fascial chains. Don't be discouraged if it doesn't work straight away, just try again.

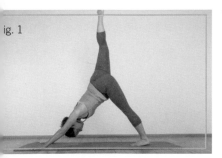
Fig. 1

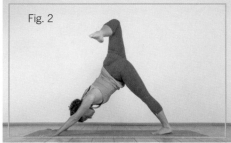
Fig. 2

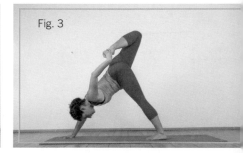
Fig. 3

Thread the needle

» Begin in tabletop position (page 26). Lift your right hand from the mat, and lay the back of the hand down. Slide your right hand through under the left arm. Slowly glide your whole arm along the mat until your right shoulder touches the floor. Lay your head on the mat at the temple, and push your weight through your shoulder into the mat. Enjoy the pleasant stretching and opening of the spiral chains in your upper body (fig. 1).
» Repeat the exercise on the other side.

Tip: By pressing the back of your hand firmly into the floor and at the same time pushing out of the mat with your supporting hand, you can increase the twist further.

Variation: "Up and down" threading

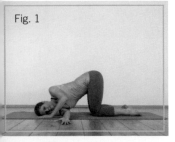
Fig. 1

» Begin in thread the needle pose. The right shoulder is placed on the mat.
» As you inhale, slowly come back up. Lift the left arm straight up from the side in a fluid movement. Turn the upper body to the right, and extend from your left hand to your right (fig. 2). As you exhale, "thread the needle" again.
» Vary how you move from breath to breath. When opening to the left, try stretching your left leg back and away from you (fig. 3). You'll feel that you can open up further. Change the angle of your shoulder by moving your arm forward or back.
» Repeat this exercise on the other side.

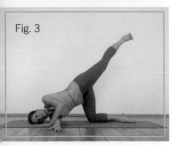
Fig. 2

Release yourself from strict movement patterns and let your creativity run free. Your fascial chains will enjoy it!

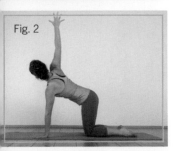
Fig. 3

Pigeon

» Begin in tabletop position (page 26). Move your left knee forward and lay the lower left leg behind your hands.
» The angle of the knee joint determines the stretch. Ideally, the lower leg should be almost parallel to the front edge of your mat. For a gentler stretch, or if you have knee problems, bend the knee more and move the heel backwards towards the left hip. The lower leg is then diagonal. Stretch your right leg backwards. The top of the foot lies on the mat (fig. 1).
» Like in thread the needle (see page 84), thread your right hand under your left arm. Lay your right shoulder on the mat (fig. 2).

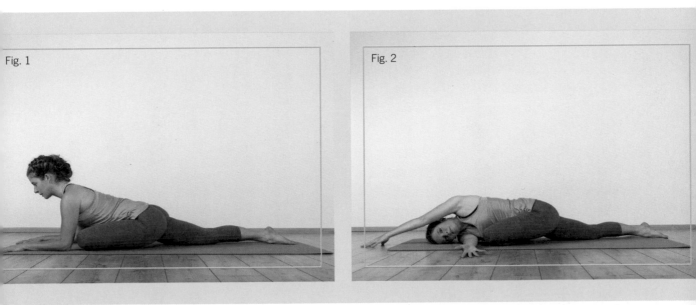

Fig. 1

Fig. 2

Relaxation for the spiral fascial chains – knee down twist

» Lie on your back and place your arms at shoulder height. Bend the right leg. With your left hand, hold the outside of your right knee. Gently pull your right knee past the centre point and over to the left side. Place your right foot on your outstretched left leg or on the floor. Release your left hand and relax your arm onto the floor. Turn your head to the right side. This extends the stretch to the whole spine (fig. 1).
» Play with the position of your right leg. Stretch the leg out and draw a circle on the floor with your foot. This changes the pull on the fascia in your lower back. Begin with small circles and let them grow bigger.
» Repeat the exercise on the other side.

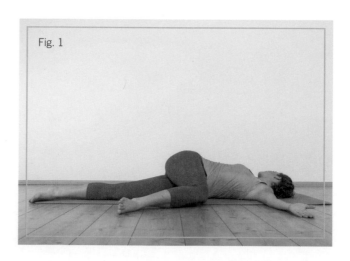

Fig. 1

Sitting half spinal twist

» Sit upright with your legs out straight in front of you. Bend your right leg to place the right foot on the outside of the left knee. As you inhale, lengthen the spine (fig. 1).
» As you exhale, turn your upper body to the right. Slowly lower the right arm and place the hand on the outside of the right thigh. With your left arm, hug your right leg. Root into the mat with both sitting bones (fig. 2).
» Repeat the exercise on the other side.

Fascia tip: Inhaling length
With each inhalation, bring a little more length to your spine. As you exhale, turn a little further into the twist.

Tip: If you find that one buttock lifts off the floor, place a meditation cushion or blanket underneath, so that you remain firmly rooted into the mat with both sitting bones.

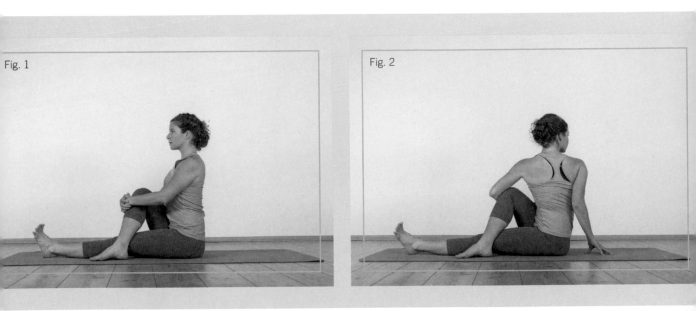

Fig. 1

Fig. 2

Arm chains

In addition to the major fascial chains that run through the body, there are also four additional chains in the arms. In yoga, the shoulders and arms play a "supporting role" in the truest sense. In our everyday lives, we are used to standing on our legs and using our hands for all kinds of movements. Sometimes, on the yoga mat, we turn things upside down. In many poses, we support ourselves or balance on our arms, and need a lot of strength and mobility.

The arms and shoulders have a very complex construction, because our shoulders – unlike our hips – are more designed for movement. There are some ten joints involved in moving the hands and arms. The shoulder area is primarily stabilised with muscles, tendons and ligaments, and has a relatively large range of motion. In order to control this, the whole muscle–ligament structure is made of branches. We can distinguish between the following fascial chains:

» Superficial front arm chain
» Deep front arm chain
» Superficial back arm chain
» Deep back arm chain.

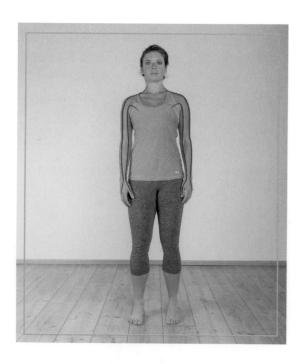

Eagle arms

» Come into an upright cross-legged position (page 24). Straighten your left arm out in front of you and lay your right arm over the left, so that the right elbow rests in the hollow of the left elbow (fig. 1).
» Twist your forearms around each other and bring the palms together. If your palms don't touch, you can bring your fingers and thumbs together. Move your arms from face height upwards, as far as is comfortable for you, and move the elbows away from your face (fig. 2). Breathe deeply and with awareness between the shoulder blades, as if you wanted to move the shoulder blades apart. Again, think in two directions. Elbows forward, shoulder blades back and out.
» Repeat on the other side.

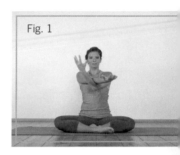

Fig. 1

Let your shoulders sink downwards. If you feel your shoulders pulling upwards, move your elbows down slightly.

Variation: Flying eagle

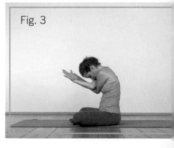

Fig. 2

» Let your eagle take off and land! As you exhale, move your elbows towards your belly button. Make sure that the movement comes mainly from your thoracic spine area – your upper back will be rounded. You will feel the stretch between your shoulder blades more intensely (fig. 3).
» As you inhale, pull the elbows up as far as possible. Your upper back straightens out again. The shoulders sink down and back, and the breastbone lifts forward (fig. 4).
» Repeat this exercise on the other side.

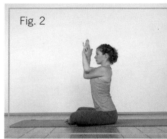

Fig. 3

Feel how the stretch in your shoulders and neck changes with just the movement of your spine (rounding and straightening) and your breathing.

Tip: Eagle is wonderfully suited to relieving tension in the shoulders and neck. Muscle tension is reduced, and the tense, knotted fascial chain is stretched out. The shoulders are said to carry a lot of weight. If we are stressed or anxious, we intuitively raise our shoulders in a protective posture, and often only notice later, when painful tension appears, how our body has reacted. In your daily life, observe when and in which situations you become a "shoulder raiser".

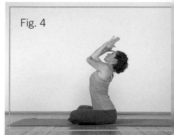

Fig. 4

Cow face

» Come into an upright cross-legged or kneeling position (pages 24 and 25). Lift your right arm straight up and allow your left arm to hang at your side. Bend both elbows. Walk your left hand up your spine, and your right hand down. Try to hold your fingertips or hands (figs 1 and 2).

» Do not abandon good posture in order to reach your hands together. If you notice that your upper body moves forward, you have a marked hollow in your lower back or your arms are pushing your head down, release your hands and increase the space between them a little. You may also work with a towel or strap (see tip).

Tip: Use a towel or strap if you can't move your hands together yet. Hold it in your right hand and then take hold of it with your left, lower hand (fig. 3).

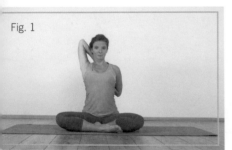

Fig. 1

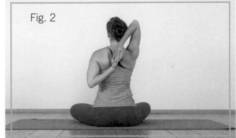

Fig. 2

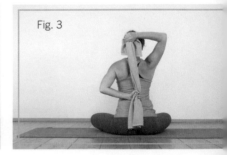

Fig. 3

Deep forward fold with clasped hands

» Start in a standing position. Clasp your hands behind your back and interlace your fingers. Lift your breastbone. Push your hands away from your body behind your back (fig. 1).

» Sink your upper body into forward fold (see page 52). The hands remain clasped behind your back. Take your arms as far up and forward as is comfortable for you. Let your whole upper body, including your head and shoulders, hang down and relax. Simply hang and let go (fig. 2).

» After seven to ten breaths, return to standing. Enjoy how open and wide your chest feels when you release your arms.

Variation: Forward fold with pulsing arms

» Pulse your arms slightly. Begin with very small movements, then becoming bigger. Relax your muscles and let your arms pulse with the strength and elasticity of the fascia alone (fig. 3).

Tip: You can also clasp your hands behind your back in many other poses in order to open your upper front body more. In deep forward fold, gravity has a particularly strong pull on your arms. You can also use this arm variation in exercises like child's pose (fig. 4) and seated forward fold.

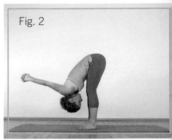

Fig. 1

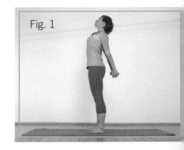

Fig. 2

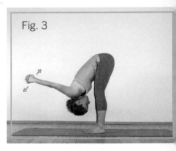

Fig. 3

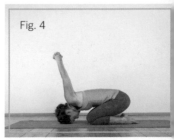

Fig. 4

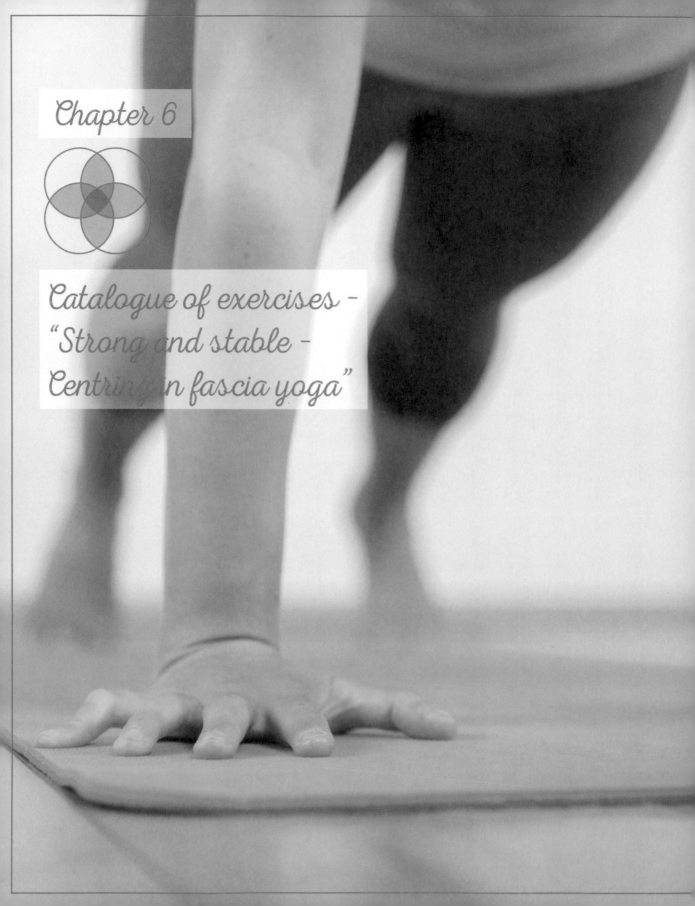

Chapter 6

Catalogue of exercises – "Strong and stable – Centring in fascia yoga"

In the previous chapters, you learned about the surface fascial chains. Now, we are going to look at the deep frontal fascial chain. Unlike the long surface connections, this deep inner fascial chain is less like a single rope, and more like a three-dimensional space. It is also referred to as the centre or core of the body. Take the term core a little further – it doesn't only refer to the abdominal muscles. Think of it extending from the arches of the feet up the insides of the legs to the pelvic floor, and all the way up the spine to the skull.

» The deep frontal fascial chain runs from the soles of the feet up the backs of the lower legs.
» It includes the whole inner thigh area.

» The main part goes to the hips, the pelvis and the lumbar spine.
» A secondary strand forms the pelvic floor and then leads back to the area of the thoracic spine.
» It covers all hip flexor, respiratory and abdominal muscles.
» From there, it continues through the chest and throat to the skull.

There are no movements in which it is not involved, and we cannot make any movements that aren't affected by it. It is constantly interacting with the surface fascial chains (see table).

Functions of the deep front fascial chain and their uses for fascia yoga

Function	Use for fascia yoga
Lifting the arch of the foot	Having a stable arch of the foot helps with pada bandha (page 20)
Stabilising the legs	Stable ankles and knees provide steadiness in standing poses
Supporting the lumbar spine from the front	A strong core prevents an over-arched back. The basic tension in the deep fascial chain protects us from overextending the lumbar spine area, particularly in back bends
Stabilising the chest	The chest is supported and elongated

The deep fascial chain primarily plays a supporting, stabilising role. The muscular area is mainly made up of long and persistent muscle fibres, which underline the role of fascia in creating a stable, upright posture.

Strengthening the core is one aspect of fascia yoga. The core is particularly important for grounding and centring your body – so give it your full attention during your practice.

Mountain

At first glance, mountain pose, standing straight and upright, seems like one of the easiest poses, but it is actually profound and complex. It improves posture and provides relief to the spine and hips. The whole inner core, from the soles of the feet to the skull, is activated. You were introduced to the posture in chapter 3, where it was presented as a starting position for many standing fascia yoga exercises. Mountain is the foundation of all standing positions, so I would like to give you further suggestions on how to deepen and centre.

» Begin standing upright and align yourself from your feet to your head (page 23). Activate your pada bandha (page 20). Imagine you are absorbing energy and strength from the ground through the soles of your feet. Let the energy rise up through your inner core, reaching the insides of your legs, the front of your spine and right up to the back of your head. You may wish to close your eyes and visualise your feet as roots anchoring you to the ground and absorbing energy into the body.
» Focus on your centre and feel the stability in your pelvis and upper body. Activate your abdominal muscles a little more with each exhalation.
» Lift your arms straight up. Keep your hands roughly shoulder width apart, so that it is easier to draw your shoulders away from your ears. Consciously push your feet into the floor again, while extending your fingertips up to the ceiling. Your spine becomes noticeably longer (fig. 1).

Tip: If you would like to, close your eyes and observe what happens.

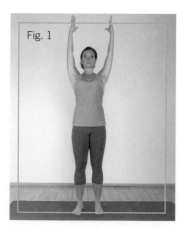

Fig. 1

Lightning bolt

Lightning bolt pose is often called chair pose, even though the position has nothing to do with sitting comfortably. Lightning bolt is an intense, strong pose that uses nearly all the muscle groups. It primarily activates the thighs and shoulders/back. These areas may at first not seem to be part of the deep front fascial chain, but a stable core is key to this pose.

» Start in a standing position. Bend your knees and sink your buttocks back and down. Tilt your pelvis back slightly, as if you were about to sit down on a chair. Activate your abdominal muscles by drawing your belly button inwards.
» Lift your outstretched arms forwards until they are level with your ears. Relax the area around your shoulders and neck (fig. 1).
» Think about extending your body. Imagine someone pulling your hip bones back and down. At the same time, someone is pulling your fingertips up and forward.

Tip: Transfer your weight back onto your heels to take the pressure off your knees. The legs remain parallel. Make sure that your knees don't move together or apart.

Variation: If you feel tension in your neck, move your arms further down, to shoulder level. This puts them parallel with the floor, although they remain outstretched (fig. 2).

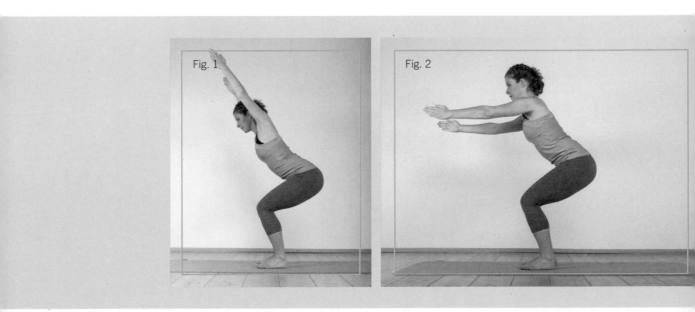

Fig. 1

Fig. 2

High plank

In dynamic yoga, high plank is often only used to transition from downward-facing dog to low plank (four-limbed staff). But high plank is a wonderful exercise for strengthening the torso, activates many of the muscles in the body and reaches the whole deep front fascial chain.

» Begin in tabletop position and align your hands properly (page 26). Straighten your legs out behind you and move onto your toes. Keep the feet hip width apart.
» Bring your heels, hips and shoulders into a single line so that you are not arching towards the ceiling or the floor (fig. 1).
» Firmly activate the thigh and abdominal muscles in order to keep the core strong and straight, like a plank of wood. Actively press away from the floor with your hands. Draw your shoulders away from your ears.

Tip: Instead of tabletop position, you can also come into high plank from downward-facing dog (page 54). From down dog, slide your upper body forwards until your shoulders are over your wrists. Then align your body in plank.

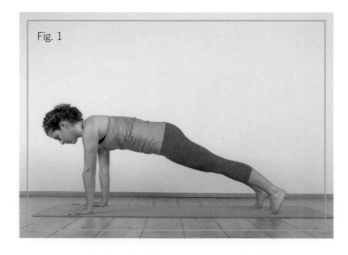

Fig. 1

Low plank

Low plank is also called the "four-limbed staff" in yoga. To an observer, the body floats above the ground, light as a feather, straight and sturdy like a staff. The hands and feet are the four supporting limbs. When practising, you will notice that this pose requires a lot of tension in the body, and you may not feel as light as a feather at first! Don't be discouraged, keep practising. Ease will come.

» Begin in high plank (page 96). Bend your elbows and sink your upper body down slowly. Your elbows stay close to your body, directly over the wrists. Lower your shoulders until they are in line with your elbows.
» The whole body remains strong and stable, and you maintain tension in the thighs and torso. In the final position, your whole body forms a line parallel to the mat (fig. 1).

Tip: Pay attention to your shoulders! Don't lower your upper body too far. The shoulders should be level with the elbows. There is a right angle between your upper and lower arms. The elbows are always at an angle of at least 90° (fig. 2). If you are not sure, film yourself in low plank or ask someone for feedback.

Variation: Place your knees on the mat and then bend your elbows to lower your upper body (fig. 3). This places much less weight on your arms, thus relieving the wrists and lower back. Make sure your torso and legs remain active! This somewhat easier variation is also a great way to prepare for the version with straight knees.

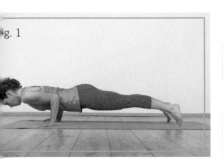

Fig. 1

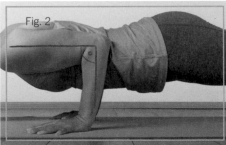

Fig. 3

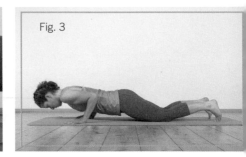

Fig. 2

Side plank

We have already got to know two core-strengthening arm-supported poses with high and low plank (pages 96 and 97). Until now, you have always kept both hands and both feet on the mat to support yourself. In side plank, you hold yourself up on one hand. This means it also challenges your balance. With a strong core, you can really master this pose.

» Begin in high plank (page 96). Turn your feet so that the outer edge of your right foot and the inner edge of your left foot are touching the mat. Release your left hand from the mat and open your whole body to the left.
» Stretch your left arm upwards. Align your left shoulder over your right shoulder.
» In addition to your stabilising abdominal muscles, activate the lateral and oblique abdominal muscles. This will allow you to lift your hips further (fig. 1).
» Return to high plank and turn to the right side.

Tip: Consciously keep the shoulder of the supporting arm rolled back, so that you do not sink into your shoulder joint.

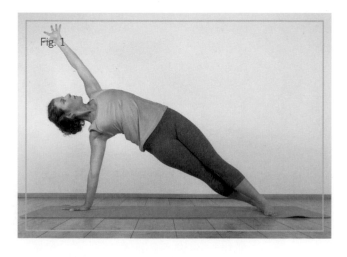

Fig. 1

Boat

Boat builds strength in all layers of the abdominal muscles, and is therefore a great pose for the deep front fascial chain. Technically, boat is a balance, as you balance your whole body on your sitting bones. As boat is a very challenging pose and can strain your lower back if your abdominal muscles are weak and if you push yourself too far, you should pay attention to your own limits. For this reason, I have also included an easier variation.

» Begin sitting on the mat. Bend your legs. Lean your upper body backwards slightly until your feet lift off the mat. Straighten your knees, bringing your feet up to approximately eye level. Your body forms a V.
» Straighten your arms, parallel to the floor. Lift your sternum and allow your shoulders to relax and slide down the spine (fig. 1).
» Hold the balance on your sitting bones. Your whole core is activated by the act of balancing.

Tip: Pull your toes back and press the insides of the balls of your feet together, with your heels moving away from each other slightly. This includes the inner thigh muscles in the pose.

Variation 1: To make the pose easier, bend your legs. This shortens the pressure lever, and the abdominal and back muscles have less weight to support (fig. 2).

Variation 2: To take the pose further, try half-boat. For this, lower your upper body and legs at the same time, until your body is almost in a straight line parallel to the floor. Your shoulders and legs remain lifted. Direct your gaze forwards to your toes (fig. 3). If you feel any pain or pressure in your lower back, return to the other variations of boat.

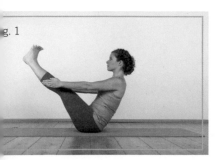

Fig. 2

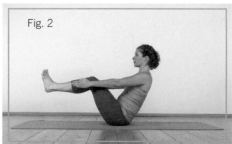

g. 1

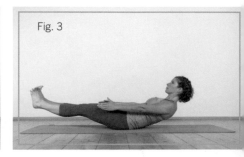

Fig. 3

Windscreen wipers

Windscreen wipers is not a traditional yoga pose. But it is a key part of fascia yoga, as it strengthens and stabilises the whole core.

» Lie on your back. Extend your legs vertically towards the ceiling. Place your arms to the sides with your palms towards the floor.
» Pull the toes towards you and press the insides of your big toes together. Tense your inner thighs. At the same time, activate your abdominal muscles and press your lower back firmly into the mat.
» As you exhale, lower your legs to the right side, keeping them together (fig. 1). As you inhale, return to centre. With your next exhalation, repeat on the left. Always keep your torso aligned to avoid shifting your lower back.

Tip: If keeping your legs straight is too intense, this pose also works with bent legs (fig. 2).

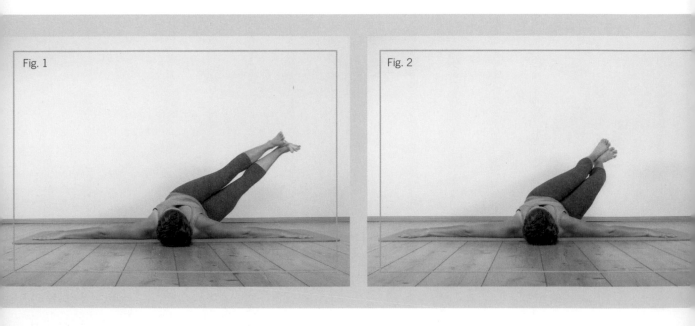

Fig. 1

Fig. 2

Tree

Tree epitomises many balance exercises. All one-legged standing poses are excellent for activating the deep front fascial chain in a playful way. The more stable your core, the stronger the roots of your tree will be. In addition to strengthening the body, tree also teaches balance and concentration.

» Stand in a straight and upright position. Lift your right leg. Hold your lower leg just under the knee and pull it towards your upper body.
» Hold your right ankle with your right hand and bring the sole of your right foot to the inner thigh of your left leg. Press your foot into your thigh, while pressing your thigh into your foot. This creates tension, which keeps you stable.
» Make sure that both hip bones are facing forwards. Open your right knee as far as possible to the side.
» Activate your abdominal muscles and lift your arms upwards (fig. 1).
» Focus on a specific point, bringing your whole awareness to it.
» Repeat the exercise on the other side.

Activate the thigh muscles of the supporting leg and straighten the knee. If your supporting leg is straight, you are mainly balancing with your ankle, rather than your knee.

Tip: No false pride. It's not about getting your foot as high as you can. It's much more important to keep your balance and open the hips. If you are having a wobbly day, place your foot on the inside of your lower leg (fig. 2) or place your toes on the floor (fig. 3).

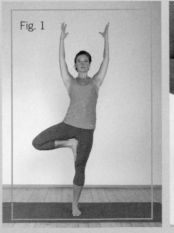
Fig. 1

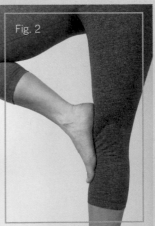
Fig. 2

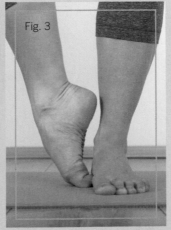
Fig. 3

Relaxation for the deep front fascial chain – tortoise

Tortoise and garland are hip-opening poses that stretch the inner thighs and relax the core.

» Sit on the mat with your legs out in front of you. Bend your knees slightly. The knees fall out to the sides, so that the soles of the feet face each other.
» Move your hands out under the knees and then place your hands on the tops of the feet.
» Round your back and roll into yourself. Holding your feet allows you to move your shoulder blades far apart (fig. 1).

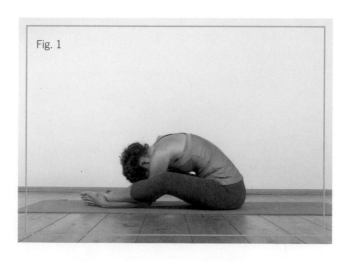

Fig. 1

Garland

» Begin standing upright, and place the feet mat width apart. The toes point slightly outwards.
» Bend your knees and sink your buttocks down as far as possible.
» Bring your elbows to the insides of your knees and hold your hands in prayer position in front of your heart (fig. 1).
» The feet stay flat on the floor.

Tip: Bring a little movement into the pose by releasing your arms and using them to explore the space around you. Transfer your weight from one foot to the other and move freely with your upper body.

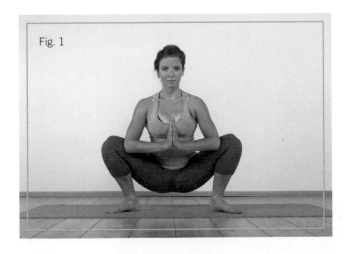

Fig. 1

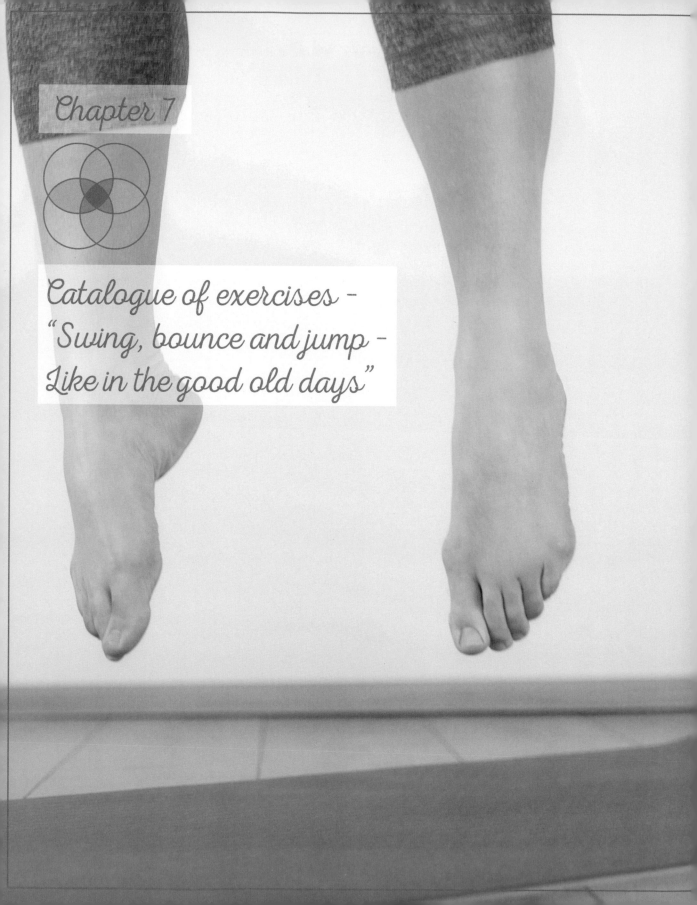

Chapter 7

Catalogue of exercises – "Swing, bounce and jump – Like in the good old days"

Swinging, bouncing, jumping and rocking – all familiar ways of moving! I'm sure you're asking yourself what they have to do with fascia yoga. A great deal! These elastic movements, which have long been some of the basic movements used in gymnastics and dancing, keep our fascial network flexible and supple.

Take a look at the animal world. Have you ever seen a kangaroo jump? Their bounding gait allows them to cover twelve metres in a single leap and to jump two metres high! Such jumps would not be possible with muscle strength alone. Studies have shown that fascia in kangaroos' legs is taut, like elastic bands. It is prestressed, so the energy is released at the moment of the jump. The force of the jump doesn't come from the muscles, but from the fascia. They work together, hand in hand. Today, we know that the human fascia has a memory potential identical to the fascia of animals like kangaroos and gazelles.

But don't worry! Fascia yoga isn't about becoming a long jumper. Bouncing, jumping and swinging are used in fascia yoga to harness the "catapult effect" of the fascia.

Fascia as elastic bands

Imagine your fascia as an elastic band that can be pulled to many times its original length. When you let go, it returns to its original form. This is thanks to the collagen (stability) and elastin (flexibility) that make up the tissue. Releasing the fascia also releases energy. When you stretch and release an elastic band, you know the force with which it springs back. We can use this energy in our movements to make them more "economical" and thus make our bodies more efficient. If our fascia is healthy and elastic, this stretching and releasing works well. But if our fascia has lost suppleness or is "sticking", the catapult effect cannot work as effectively.

But what exactly is the difference between bouncing and swinging? When does jumping stop and springing start? How do I use the catapult effect? I have organised this "catalogue of elastic exercises" according to the various forms of movement. Begin with the easiest exercises from the bouncing and swinging sections to warm up and prepare the body. These forms of movement are particularly good for this, and the body should already be warmed up before you try the jumps and prestressing exercises. With a warm, well-prepared body, you will feel the "catapult effect" more clearly.

Let's bounce!

Bouncing is a rhythmic, elastic up-and-down movement of the body, in which no active muscle tensing takes place. If the bouncing movements are performed in the legs, at least one foot remains in constant contact with the floor. There is no "flying" like with jumping and springing. When you bounce, your muscles are only involved passively. It is primarily the fascial network – the muscle fascia, tendons and ligaments – that creates the movement. The challenge with bouncing is in carrying out the movement rhythmically and with ease, without tensing any muscles. Try it out for yourself!

Stand upright on both feet and start to lift and lower your heels rhythmically. Your heels should not touch the floor (fig. 1). Then try lifting one foot from the floor and bouncing on one leg (fig. 2). How does the bouncing feel? Have you found your rhythm? Move with awareness!

In the following exercises, you use the fascia's capacity for memory in small bouncing movements. Bounce and pulse smoothly and gently.

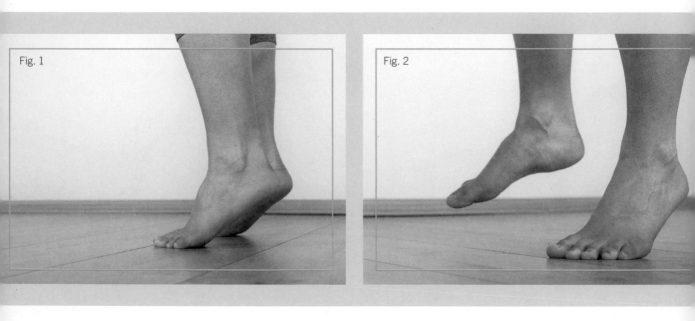

Fig. 1

Fig. 2

Dancing dog

Bouncing the upper body: Come into downward-facing dog (page 54). Open your shoulders with awareness and push your sternum far back between your arms. Repeat this movement until you feel your upper body becoming softer. From this controlled motion of pushing back the upper body, you can gradually develop a soft bouncing backwards between your arms (fig. 1).

Bouncing heels: Bend your knees slightly. Begin to very gently pulse the heels, and let the pulsing movements gradually grow bigger (fig. 2). Make sure to keep your upper body long and extended.

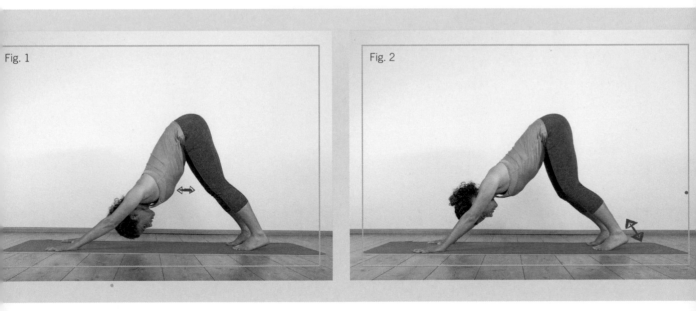

Fig. 1

Fig. 2

Palm in the wind

» Begin in crescent, leaning to the left (page 72). Your right arm lifts up and leans to the left.
» Bring small bouncing movements into the side bend. Gradually increase the intensity of your bounce. With your left hand, feel how your ribs move apart like compartments, and the muscles between your ribs are loosened and stretched (fig. 1).
» Repeat this exercise on the other side.

Fascia tip: Cross your legs
When you lean to the right, place your left foot behind the right (fig. 2). This moves the tension further over the outside of your hip into the leg, down to the ankle. Note that this variation requires more balance.

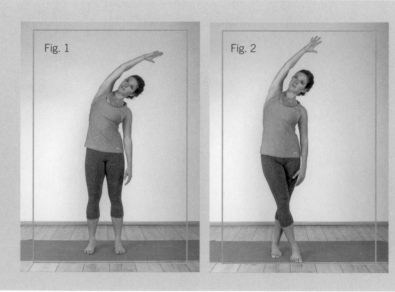

Pulsing forward fold

» Come into standing forward fold (page 52). Use your hands to hold your elbows and let your upper body hang down (fig. 1).
» Begin to gently pulse your upper body. As you pulse, move from one side to the other to vary the movement. Keep your knees bent slightly, taking the tension from the backs of your legs and concentrating the stretch in the lower back fascia.
» Keep your movements small and pulsing; avoid large movements.

Tip: The broad lumbar fascia covers the whole lower back and has a huge number of sensory receptors – including pain receptors.

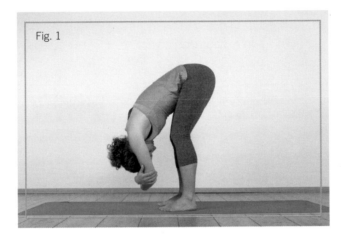

Fig. 1

Dynamic swinging

When pulsing movements become bigger, they can be described as swinging movements. Swinging movements comprise three main components. They begin with a countermovement, followed by the actual swing, and the movement ends with a bracing action, which can in turn be a new countermovement. In swinging, the catapult effect is used, which requires the inclusion of the fascial structures.

Gravity is used to drive the motion in the swinging phase. Let yourself go completely in this phase. The swinging exercises are perfect for gently increasing your range of motion and developing a feel for how your body tenses and relaxes, something we often lose sight of.

Lightning bolt and forward fold

» Inhale and come into lightning bolt (page 95). Bring tension into your arms, torso and legs (fig. 1).

» As you exhale, allow your upper body to relax fully and fall into a deep forward fold (fig. 2). This stretches your thick lumbar fascia – but only if your back is relaxed and rounded as you hang forwards. Always keep your knees bent (fig. 3).

» Stay in forward fold for only a short time. Use the tensile force from stretching your lumbar fascia to swing back to lightning bolt as you breathe in. Create tension again, straightening your back and arms.

With this exercise, you will feel the shift between tension and relaxation wonderfully. In lightning bolt, your body must be strong and work against gravity. As you swing downwards you can release and enjoy the falling sensation. Move more intensely at first to internalise the release. In other words, swing freely with no muscle tension.

Fascia tip: Small jump at the tipping point
As you reach the lowest point of your downward swing – the point at which you start moving upwards again – release the swinging energy with a small jump. As you jump, your upper body hangs down (fig. 4). As soon as your feet touch the ground again (it's only a small jump), the upper body swings back up again. Land softly and gently.

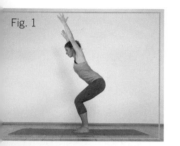
Fig. 1

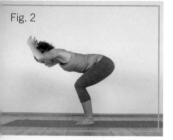
Fig. 2

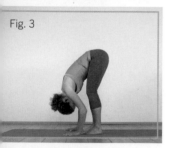
Fig. 3

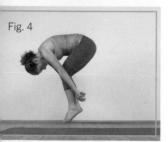
Fig. 4

Standing straight angle pose with an upper-body swing

Standing straight angle pose stretches the whole back of the body. The wide position of the legs also allows you to reach parts of the spiral fascial chains, and the lower back in particular. Enjoy the swinging phase, the sensation of falling and letting go.

» Place your feet approximately one metre apart, a little more or less depending on the length of your legs. Your toes point forwards so that your feet are parallel. Roll your upper body downwards until you can touch the floor with your hands.
» Gently swing your upper body from one foot to the other. Let your head, shoulders and arms hang down, fully relaxed (figs 1 and 2). Gradually increase the size of your movements.

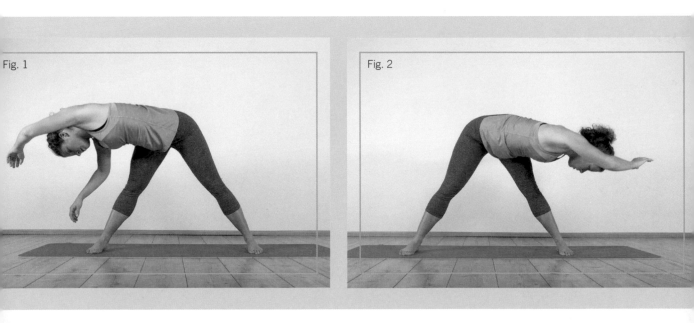

Fig. 1

Fig. 2

Leg swing

This exercise and the following, figure of eight, bring movement to your hips and help you to sway them smoothly. Both exercises are good for warming up and opening the hips, providing an excellent way to prepare for standing poses such as tree. Let's swing!

» Stand upright, and lift your left foot a short distance from the floor. Create stability in your right leg. Swing your left leg forwards and backwards evenly (fig. 1).
» Let the movement grow bigger. Now we add the fascial component: the leg swings back until your hip is completely straight (fig. 2). The fascia at the front of the hip is completely stretched, and the leg then springs forwards as if by itself.
» As the leg moves forward, it comes up as far as your mobility allows (fig. 1). As soon as the back of your leg is tensed, the leg automatically comes back.
» After one to two minutes, change onto your left leg and swing the right leg. Swing it out and find your rhythm.

Tip: You may find it easier to swing more loosely standing on a raised platform (fig. 3). A stack of two or three books will be enough to make your leg swing long and straight.

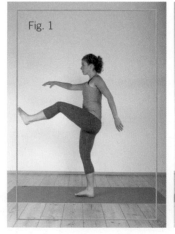
Fig. 1

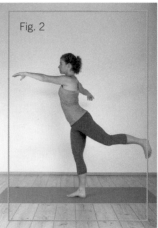
Fig. 2

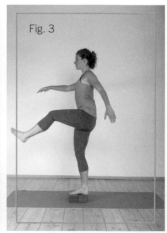
Fig. 3

Figure of eight

» Stand upright, and lift your right foot a short distance from the floor. Create stability in your left leg. Bend the right leg. Use your right knee to draw a sideways figure of eight in the air. This rotates the hip inwards and outwards (figs 1 and 2). Start with slow, controlled movements to get a feeling of the sequence.

» Bring a little more swing to your movement. The range of motion of the swing is much smaller than with leg swing. It is more a matter of finding your rhythm – the balance between control and release.

Tip: Hold on. Swinging your leg means that your centre of gravity is moving constantly. This can lead to you being rather wobbly! Hold onto something stable (the edge of a door, or a wall, etc.). This allows you to focus all your attention on the swinging motion.

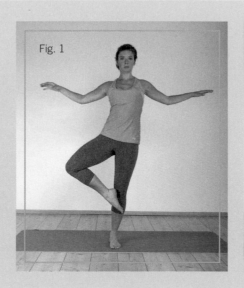
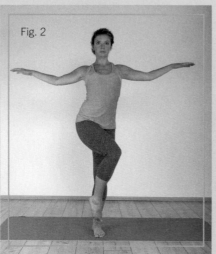

Fig. 1

Fig. 2

Flat back with swinging arms

Swinging your arms helps to loosen the shoulder area, which is often tense. If you extend the swinging movement to your upper body by rotating from one side to the other, you can enjoy a twist in your spine.

» Begin in flat back position (fig. 1). The upper body is parallel to the floor, the head remains in line with the cervical spine, and the torso is active and tensed. Bend your knees slightly, making it easier to keep your back straight. Your arms point forwards.
» From this position, swing your arms in opposite directions, forwards and back, from the shoulders. The movement gradually grows bigger (fig. 2).
» Let the swinging of your arms move into your upper body. Twist your upper body to the open side with your arms. As your arms swing past each other under your body, go with the movement with your upper body, letting it fall down. As your arms lift and move apart, lift your upper body a little too. The swinging of your arms and upper body remains loose, dynamic and easy (fig. 3). Find your own rhythm.

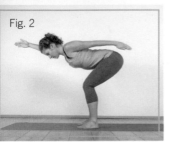
Fig. 1

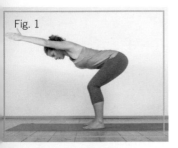
Fig. 2

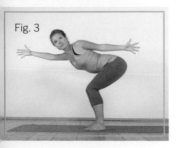
Fig. 3

Elastic

Jumping and springing exercises are brought together in one group of exercises. The only difference between springing and jumping lies in the length of the "flying" phase. A spring is a small jump, and a jump is a big spring. With both movements, both feet (or hands!) leave the floor for a moment. In jumping, the muscles and fascia work hand in hand. First, your body is pre-tensioned, for example by bending your knees (muscle activity – the fascia is already pre-tensioned). Then, from bending your knees you spring like a kangaroo up and along (figs 1 and 2). The energy comes from both your muscles and your pre-tensioned fascia, which releases your saved energy and thus supports the muscles.

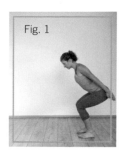

Fig. 1

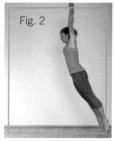

Fig. 2

In springing, the muscles play much less of a role in the movement. The muscle fascia and tendons take on most of the work. For fascia yoga, it therefore makes sense to use small springing movements rather than big jumps. Try the following exercises and remember how much you used to love springing and jumping as a child! Over the years, our bodies learn basic forms of movement. In fascia yoga, you return to a childlike state, with the goal of recovering elasticity.

Tip: Grab a skipping rope and start jumping in all directions (fig. 3).

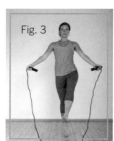

Fig. 3

Big jumps

Don't be afraid of jumping. Fascia acts as a shock absorber in our body: it transfers external forces throughout the whole body, so that the impact is not focused on one joint. This mechanism needs to be trained, as your fascia is constantly required to perform this function in your everyday life.

Springing cat

Our shoulder area was developed for a variety of movements. Throwing spears to hunt animals, cutting wood to make fires ... Unfortunately, today our lives require such movements less and less. So you need to be creative! Imagine you're a cat, playing wildly with a ball of wool. This exercise is wonderfully diverse and activates our fascial chains around the shoulders and torso. Use the supple, easy movements of a cat as your guide.

» Begin in tabletop position (page 26). Bend your elbows slightly and push yourself up from the mat. Gently cushion the landing of your hands by bending your elbows.
» Start your next "spring". This time, spread your hands further apart (fig. 1). With each new spring, change the placement of your hands and their position, as well as your centre of gravity, slightly (figs 2 and 3). Try springing more to the right, then more to the left. Come further forward, or cross your hands in front of you. Be creative and curious in finding new movements.
» Make sure that your springing movements are always soft, like a rubber ball. If, after repeating this a few times, the exercise feels more like push-ups, this means your muscles are working too hard.

Tip: To warm up your upper body and spine in preparation, I recommend the "wild cat" exercise (page 60).

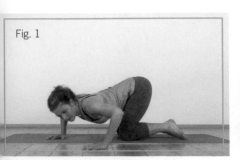
Fig. 1

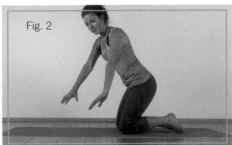
Fig. 2

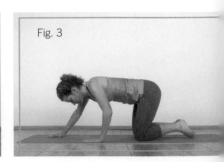
Fig. 3

Springing dog

Transitioning from downward-facing dog (page 54) to plank or forward fold as gracefully as possible is a challenge in the dynamic sun salutation. In fascia yoga, you can make this transition in a way that is good for your fascia by springing or even jumping.

From dog to high plank

» Begin as if performing dancing dog (page 107), gently pulsing your heels. Your heels move up and down at the same time. The pulsing gets bigger and you begin to spring on the spot, with both feet leaving the floor for a short moment. Gently cushion the springing with your whole body. Your body moves elastically with each spring (fig. 1).
» Slowly spring backwards, with lots of small movements, into high plank (page 96, fig. 2). Then slowly spring back to downward-facing dog.
» Repeat this change in positions four to five times.

From dog to forward fold

» Here, spring forwards, with lots of little springs, from downward-facing dog into a deep forward fold. The feet move towards the hands (figs 3 and 4). It isn't a problem if you can't spring your feet all the way forward. Walk the last few centimetres with both feet.

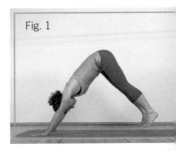

Fig. 1

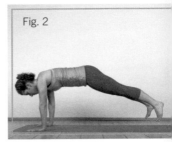

Fig. 2

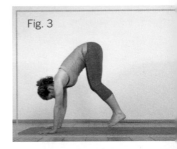

Fig. 3

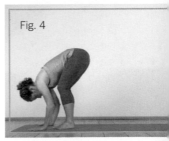

Fig. 4

Jumping from dog to garland

When jumping from dog, your Achilles tendons are pre-tensioned. This energy then releases when you jump. Even if the length you can jump isn't quite enough to reach your hands at first, try again and have courage. Enjoy the feeling of standing on your hands for just a moment as your feet leave the floor.

» Begin in downward-facing dog (page 54). Bend your knees a little more, so your heels lift up. Stretch your upper body as far as you can, and push your buttocks back and up. Direct your gaze forwards to your hands and look at the points to the right and left outside your hands. These are where your feet should land (fig. 1).
» Push off from the mat using your legs. Straighten your legs like a catapult. During your jump, your buttocks are drawn upwards (fig. 2). Your feet land outside your hands to the right and left. After landing, lower your buttocks towards the ground (fig. 3). Leave your hands on the floor, and come back to downward-facing dog with a jump or two big steps.
» Repeat this exercise five to six times.

Never land with your legs straight. With bent legs, you can absorb the effects of the impact on the body much better.

Tip: You can also use jumping dog as a way to transition into forward fold, including it in the sun salutation. In downward-facing dog, fix your gaze on your hands in front of you on the mat, and then place your feet directly behind your hands, rather than outside them.

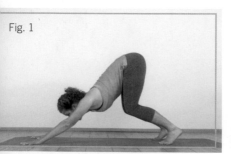
Fig. 1

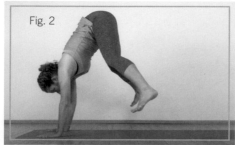
Fig. 2

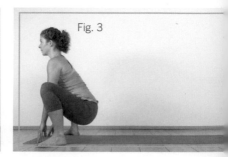
Fig. 3

Frog jump

The frog jump in fascia yoga works just like a frog jump in nature. The squatting position pre-tenses the thighs and the Achilles tendons. As you catapult upwards, the energy stored is used in the fascia and the strength of the muscles is used to spring as high as possible into the air. Don't try this exercise without warming up first.

» Come into garland (fig. 1).
» Extend your legs and use your strength to push off the floor. The whole body extends when you are in the air (fig. 2).
» Land back in garland, and gently cushion the jump.
» Repeat the jump five to six times or until you feel your legs losing strength.

Tip: What if you changed perspective? Spiral as you jump upwards, and land facing the opposite direction. Turn twice on your own axis and come back to facing forwards.

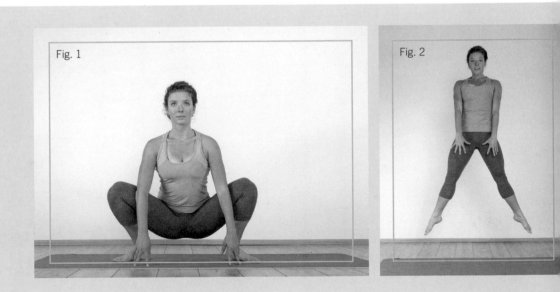

Fig. 1

Fig. 2

Jumping lunge

» Begin in high lunge (page 26). The right leg is in front, and the left leg stretched out behind you. Begin to gently pulse the hips up and down. Direct your focus to your left hip bone, which moves up and down as you pulse (fig. 1). The left hip flexor muscles gradually become softer. Carefully lift the upper body a little more, so that you feel the stretch in the whole left side of your body.

» After pulsing four or five times, change legs with a jump (fig. 2). Your left foot comes forward and the right leg is now stretched back behind you (fig. 3). Pulse again here, then change.

Tip: Use two yoga blocks or two books to support you and make the exercise easier. Place your hands on these platforms so the distance for your arms to reach a steady surface is not as far. You can stay more upright in your upper body, and your legs have more space to switch places under your body (fig. 4).

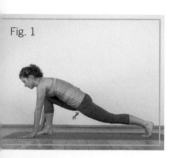

Fig. 1

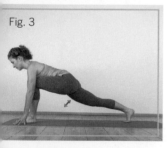

Fig. 2

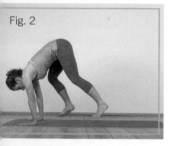

Fig. 3

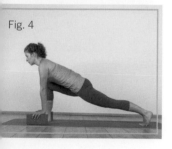

Fig. 4

Like a catapult

To make use of the catapult effect of fascia, individual movements are initiated with a countermovement in the other direction. You can imagine this principle like an arrow being loaded in a bow. The fascia, which is pre-tensioned by the movement in the opposite direction, is represented by the bow. The tension releases in the actual direction of the movement. We can take mountain and forward fold as examples from fascia yoga (you've already seen both of these poses). The actual target movement is the deep forward fold. By aligning in mountain with a slight back bend, the whole front fascial chain is tensed. As soon as the bow has enough tension, i.e. you are far enough into the back bend, you release the tension by swinging your upper body forwards. This makes the upper body the arrow, which is "shot" forwards by the active pre-tensing of the body. Getting the timing right is key to ensuring that the movement requires as little muscle tension as possible. Try it out! The aim is to relax the body and let go.

First control, then let go and enjoy

For all of the following exercises, I recommend first practising the sequence of movements slowly, in a controlled way and without swinging. After four to five repetitions, gradually let go in order to have the desired ease, rhythm and momentum as you flow through the movement. This has the advantage of giving you greater certainty about the movements, so that you can then switch off your mind and simply enjoy the flow of the movement. You'll also become more aware of the difference between control and release.

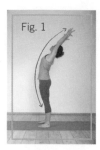

Fig. 1

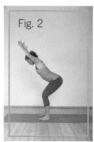

Fig. 2

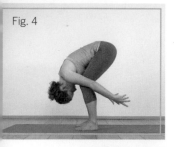

Fig. 3

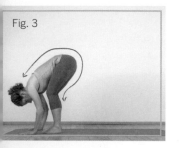

Fig. 4

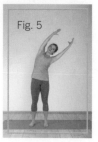

Fig. 5

From mountain to forward fold

» Begin in mountain pose (page 94). As you inhale, lean a little further back with your upper body. This pre-tenses your whole front body (fig. 1).

» As you exhale, let your upper body swing down (fig. 2). Your arms fall forwards and down (fig. 3). When your upper body has come down, swing your arms past your legs (fig. 4). Use the swinging of your arms to propel yourself back up, using as little energy as you can.

» First practise this sequence of movements with control, gradually letting go until you are swinging your whole upper body freely and loosely.

It is not only your arms that provide the drive to move back upwards. In forward fold, your back is briefly and dynamically pre-stretched. This fascia energy also releases as you move upwards. Imagine that in mountain pose, your whole front body is stretched like an elastic band. At the moment you swing your body downwards, you release the elastic band – and it quickly snaps together again. In forward fold, the back of your body is the stretched elastic band. And here, again, it snaps together as you release – bringing your upper body back upwards.

Tip: In fascia yoga, don't cling to rigid ideas about how an exercise should look. If you want to bend your legs more as you swing, then do it! If you want to stretch your upper body to the left or the right, do it (fig. 5)! Open your arms further? No problem, go for it! The exercises come to life with your ideas.

Forward fold to pulsing upright

» Begin in forward fold (page 52). Loosen up a little, so that your shoulders, neck and head hang down, fully relaxed.

» Start making small pulsing movements, like in the pulsing forward fold (page 109). Let the movement grow bigger, your upper body moving up and down like a rubber ball. The whole upper body hangs, relaxed, so that the movement comes mainly from fascia (fig. 1). You'll probably already be able to feel how your upper body is catapulted upwards as if automatically.

» Pulse three times while leaning down in order to pre-tense the lower back fascia. After the third time, pulse back to an upright position (fig. 2).

» Then drop back towards the floor, pulse again three times and come back up.

You should not do this exercise if you have high blood pressure, cardiovascular problems or are pregnant. If during the exercise you feel that constantly moving up and down doesn't agree with you, pause for a moment and then move on to the next exercise.

Variation: Of course, you can also include the pulsing upward movement in all other forward folds. Standing straight angle pose (page 111) is particularly suited to this, as you can pulse all the way back with your arms through your legs, making the pre-tensing of the back fascia much more significant (fig. 3).

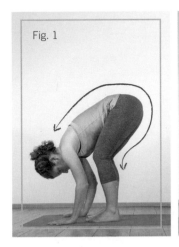
Fig. 1

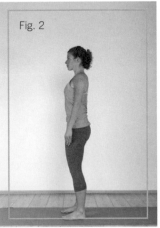
Fig. 2

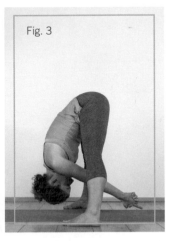
Fig. 3

Swinging warrior

» Begin in warrior pose (page 62). The right leg is forward. Bring awareness to stabilising your core by drawing your belly button inwards, actively stretching your back leg and centring your legs in relation to your core, as you need a steady starting position.

» Now lift your left arm up and stretch as far as you can upwards. With your upper body, come into a slight back bend. Tilt your pelvis backwards slightly. You will feel the tension increasing in your left hip flexor and thigh. Your left arm, upper body and left leg form a long curve, like a C (fig. 1).

» From this pre-tensing of the front body, let your upper body fall down and forwards as you exhale. Your arm also swings down past your left leg. Round your back and bend your left knee to remove all the tension from your left side (fig. 2).

» As you breathe in, come back up, stretching up and back again.

» Repeat the swinging action for seven to eight breaths, then change to the other side. Swing up and down without pausing. As you inhale you stretch upward, as you exhale you drop down.

Tip: This exercise encourages balance. As you can't fix your eyes on a specific point, it is very difficult to stay balanced. Hold onto a chair or windowsill with your free hand so that you can concentrate on letting go. It may also help to spread your feet a little wider apart. You will be much more stable with your feet approximately two hand widths apart.

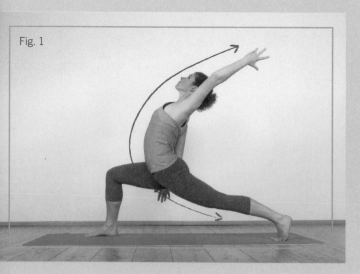

Fig. 1

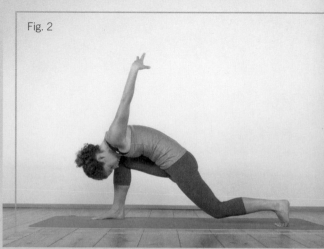

Fig. 2

Rolling plow

» Sitting on the mat, pull your legs in towards you, rounding your back and making yourself as small as possible (fig. 1).
» Now roll backwards over your rounded spine and bring your legs over your head into plow (page 56, fig. 2).
» Without pausing, roll back up and stretch your legs out in front of you. Go with the swing and stretch your upper body forwards over your legs in a forward fold (fig. 3).
» In the same way, come back again into plow. Roll back and forth a few times. You will find your own rhythm.

Always remember to consciously round your back in order to roll back and forth gently and fluidly.

Fascia tip: Vary the forward fold
You can certainly change the position of your legs – the main thing is you come into a forward fold with your upper body. Would you like to spread them wider (fig. 4)? Or maybe bend one leg and stretch the other out in front of you (fig. 5)? Perhaps stretch to the side? Would you rather move your upper body to the front or to one side? Over the straight leg or the bent leg (fig. 6)? As you can see, there are many possibilities. Your fascia loves change and new directions.

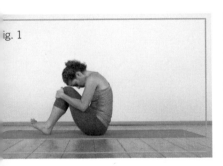

ig. 1

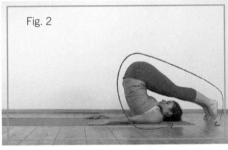

Fig. 2

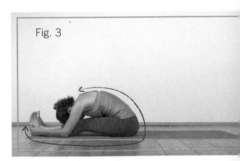

Fig. 3

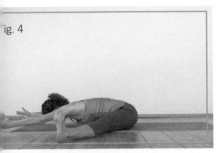

ig. 4

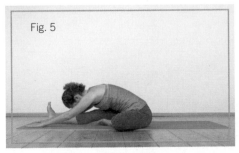

Fig. 5

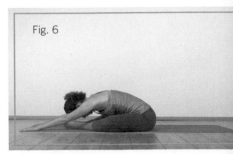

Fig. 6

Chapter 8

Catalogue of exercises –
"Body awareness with conscious breathing and relaxation"

When we talk about the five senses we use to perceive the world around us, we generally mean the eyes (seeing), nose (smelling), mouth (tasting), ears (hearing) and skin (touching). But what do we mean by body awareness, our "sense of the body"? We use it every day, in every tiny movement, but don't often pay it much attention. Sensing and being aware of movements in our body (and not only around it) form our perception of our bodies. This plays a particularly important role with regard to lack of mobility and the resulting complaints, and in psychosomatic conditions.

Proprioception – our awareness of the body

You may have already heard the term "proprioception". "Proprius" means "one's own" and "recipere" means to take or grasp. Proprioception is therefore our sense of our own body. Our proprioceptive capacities ensure that we are aware of our body and its position in space. They are responsible for how we sense our body. This perception takes place using receptors, as with the other five senses. For example, we have special receptors in the eyes that allow us to see colours. If you touch a hot stovetop, the thermoreceptors and pain receptors in your skin react and immediately send a signal to your brain: "Careful, hot, take your hand away." The brain then sends a signal to the hand muscles.

Fascia – our sixth sense

The fascial network contains around six times more sensitive nerve endings than the muscles. If we take into account all receptors, the number of fascia receptors is greater than the number of retina receptors – previously thought to be the most sensitive organ. Fascia is much more than connective parts and a means of transport! It is our most important organ for perception. The fascial network has many different types of receptors that react to different stimuli. This variety makes it clear why we use many different exercise techniques in fascia yoga. We need varied, creative movements to reach all of the receptors!

Breathing is fascia training!

Breathing is also fascia training – and breath training is a central element of fascia yoga. The diaphragm is the "motor" of our breathing, as this plate of muscle and tendons separates the abdomen from the chest. The rhythmic relaxing and contracting of this "myofascia" (muscle fascia) is what drives our inhaling and exhaling (see figure below).

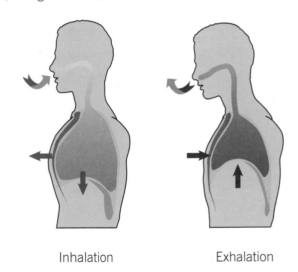

Inhalation   Exhalation

The movement of the chest when we breathe

Breathing in: The diaphragm contracts and lowers, and the outer intercostal muscles (between the ribs) are activated. This lifts the chest up and expands it. The sternum lifts up and the abdominal muscles naturally curve outwards. The lungs expand.

Breathing out: The diaphragm relaxes and curves upwards in the chest cavity. The outer intercostal muscles relax, lowering the chest. The abdominal muscles sink inwards and the lungs pull together elastically.

This rhythmic change between contraction and relaxation continuously changes the pressure on the fascia in our respiratory system – and more, because, as you know, everything forms a single unit. The aim of the following breathing exercises is to focus your attention on this contraction and relaxation, and move the body parts and organs involved as much as possible through deeper breathing.

Full yoga breathing – getting to know all breathing spaces

With full yoga breathing, you explore all three breathing spaces: abdomen, chest and collarbone. Your cells will absorb much more oxygen, as you will be using your lungs to their full capacity. With abdominal breathing, you already fill most of your lungs, but by breathing up to your collarbone, you can reach the small additional part of the tips of the lungs. Your respiratory fascial network is completely stretched in full yoga breathing, and your lungs are fully "inflated". Another positive side effect of including the chest and collarbone in your breathing is that the body is more upright as the spine is stretched.

On physical exertion, our breathing deepens naturally, as our muscles need more oxygen to cope. These mechanisms are controlled by our nervous system. But how often do we actually exert ourselves physically today? We spend more and more time sitting, both in offices and at home. This makes our breathing increasingly flat, and the oxygen supply to our body and mind (the brain requires the most oxygen) decreases significantly. Full yoga breathing is not just a tool we use in fascia yoga to stretch the respiratory fascial structures. It will also make you more efficient and help you feel refreshed – not only physically, but also mentally and spiritually.

How it works

First practise directing your breathing into one specific breathing space. Then connect all the breathing spaces together. The following describes full yoga breathing in a lying position. You can also try it sitting on a meditation cushion or a chair, or even standing.

Tip: Closing your eyes helps you be more aware and perceptive, and your senses focus fully on what is happening in your body.

Abdominal breathing

Come into a comfortable position lying on your back, and place your hands either side of your belly button. Be aware of your hands, and focus all your attention on the area around your belly button (fig. 1). Gradually begin to focus your breathing on the abdominal area. Breathe in through your nose and send your breath to your hands. Breathing out through the nose happens almost automatically – let the breath gently flow out. As you breathe in, you can feel with your hands how the abdominal wall lifts and the abdomen curves upwards. You may also feel the diaphragm dropping down and the lower parts of the lungs filling with air. As you exhale, the tension releases again. Repeat this abdominal breathing exercise for one to two minutes.

Fig. 1

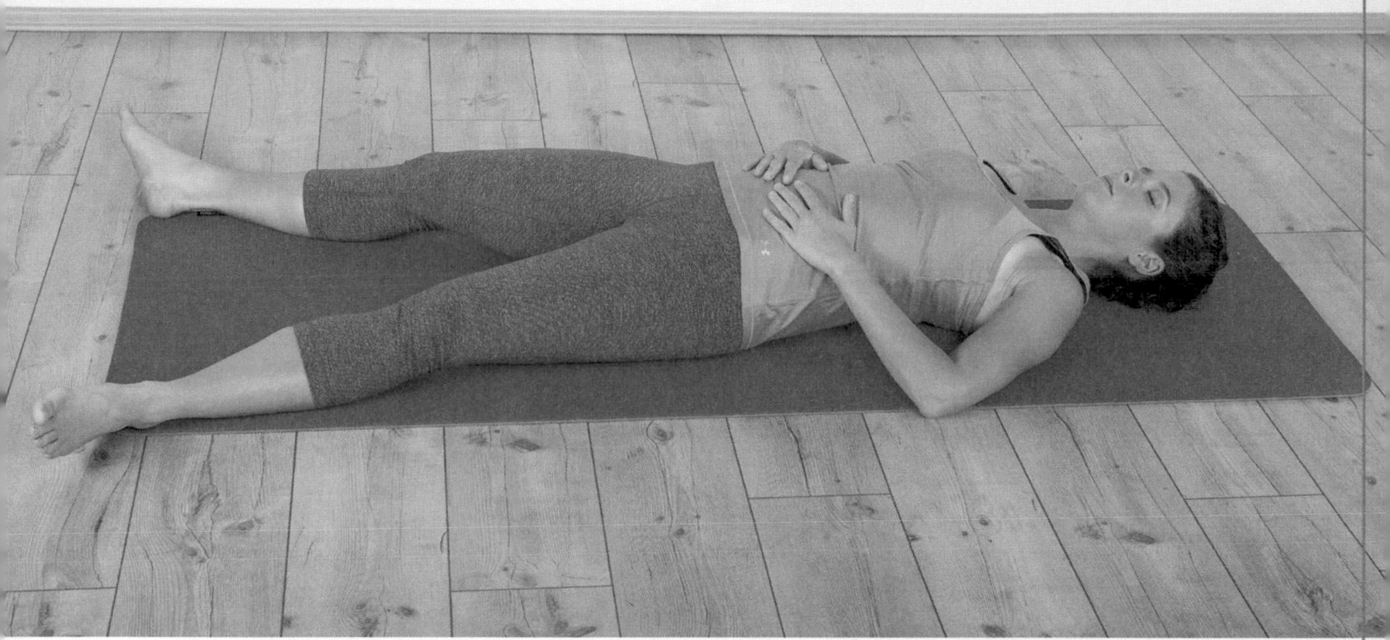

Fig. 2

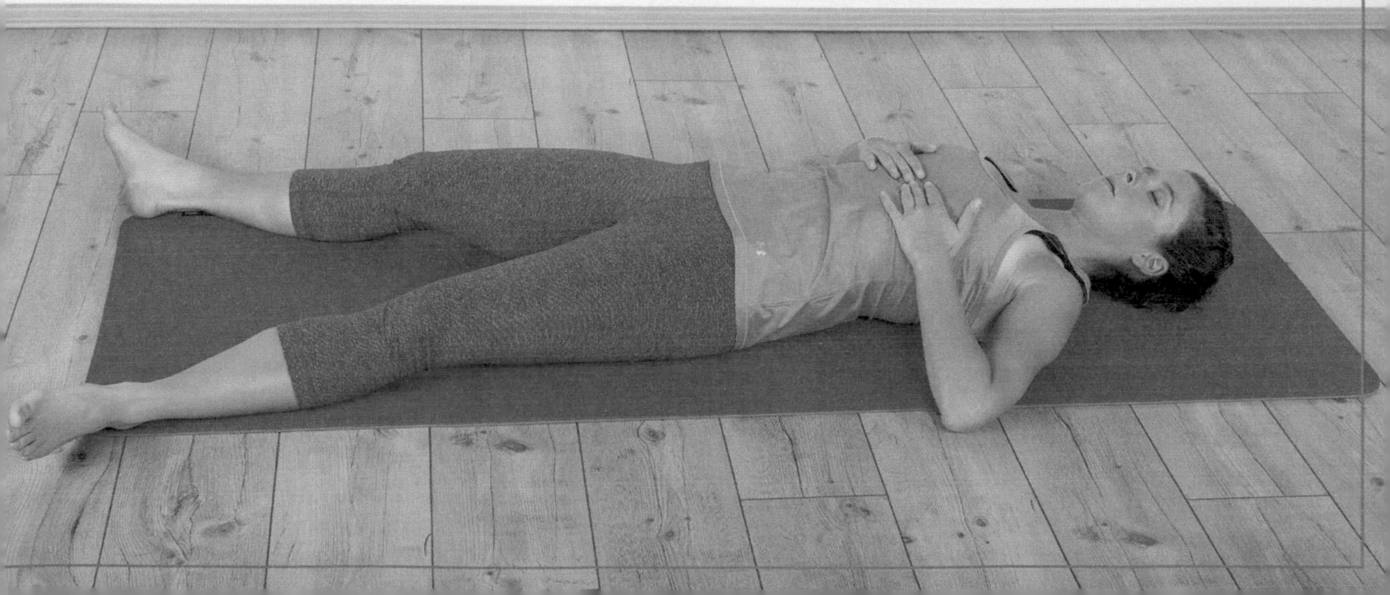

Fig. 3

Fig. 4

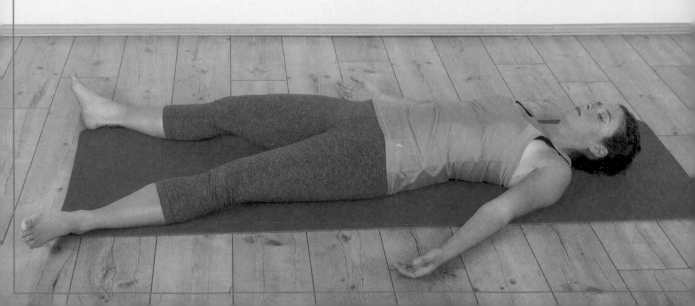

Chest breathing

Place your hands on the sides of your ribcage, so that your fingertips are pointing towards each other and touching (fig. 2). Focus all of your attention on the area under your hands. Now breathe into the chest specifically, and less into the abdomen. As you inhale, the chest stretches, the ribs are pushed apart and the middle part of the lungs can be filled with oxygen. Be aware of how your fingertips move away from each other as you inhale, and back together as you exhale. Feel the difference in comparison to abdominal breathing! Are your breaths deeper or flatter with chest breathing than with abdominal breathing? Is it easier to breathe into your abdomen or your chest?

Repeat this chest breathing exercise for one to two minutes.

Collarbone breathing

Place your hands flat on your chest, so that your fingertips touch your collarbones (fig. 3). Direct all of your attention to the area under your hands. Breathe specifically into your collarbone area. As you inhale, the collarbone lifts upwards. Let your shoulders relax into the mat and try to breathe into your abdomen and chest as little as possible. Repeat this breathing exercise for one to two minutes.

Full yoga breathing

The three breathing spaces we have just looked at are now connected in one breath. As you inhale, first the abdomen, then the chest and finally the collarbone are lifted. You exhale almost automatically. First the abdomen sinks, then the ribs are pulled together and the collarbone lowers back down. After exhaling, you inhale again, so that the breathing becomes a wavelike movement, flowing uninterrupted through the whole body (fig. 4).

Inhalation: Abdomen – Chest – Collarbone
Exhalation: Abdomen – Chest – Collarbone

Fascia tip: Fill your body with your breath, so that the whole breathing space is full of air. This moment of absolute fullness also stretches the fascial network in the respiratory organs and muscles in all directions.

Kapalabhati - boosting the diaphragm

Translated literally, this breathing exercise is called "skull-shining", and it is also known as "breath of fire". Kapalabhati clears the nose and activates prana, our "life force". This breathing technique is characterised by a strong, active exhalation and an automatic inhalation. Kapalabhati is an essential part of fascia yoga, as it strengthens the diaphragm (part of the fascia) and the muscles that help with respiration, as well as causing them to vibrate. The heart, liver and stomach are massaged by the strong, sharp exhalations. The stronger exhaling of carbon dioxide also has a cleansing effect, as toxins and acids are released from the body (see chapter 10).

Tip: Clean your nose before starting the exercise. The breathing movement is similar to blowing your nose.

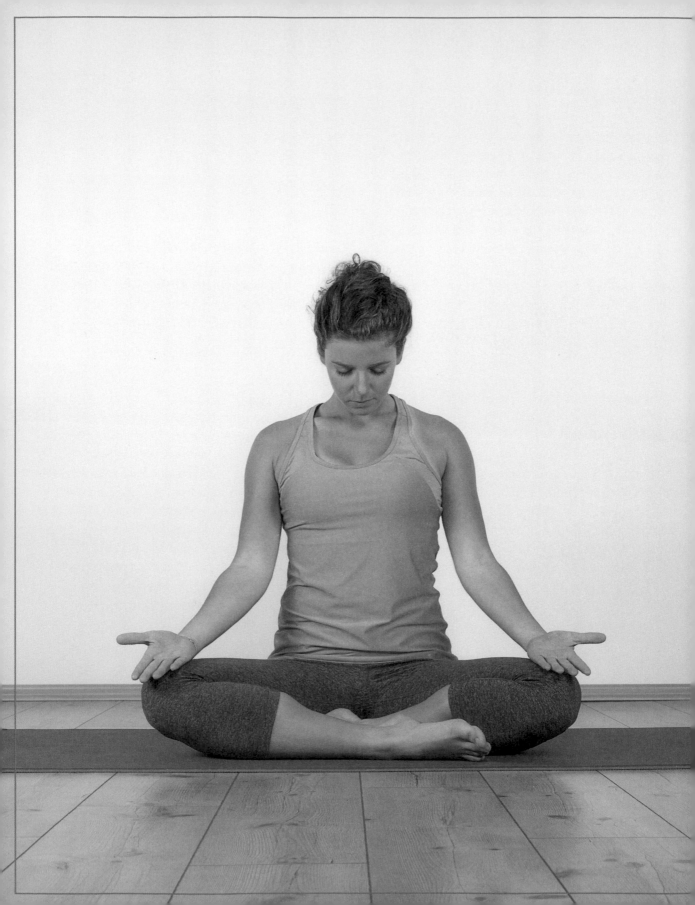

How it works

» Sitting upright, breathe in once deeply and with awareness.
» As you exhale, push the air out of your nose forcefully. The "blowing" action is very strong as a result of the abdominal wall being pulled inwards quickly and vigorously.
» When the tension in the abdomen is released, the abdominal wall expands again and fresh air flows in automatically.
» The chest does not move at all throughout the exercise.
» Begin at first at a tempo that is pleasant for you, perhaps one breath per second. Gradually speed up so that your breathing rate is up to two times faster.
» Repeat this active exhaling and passive inhaling for 20 to 30 breaths. End the exercise with a deep exhalation and then let your breathing flow freely in a relaxed manner. Be mindful. See if you feel any changes.

Repeat this breathing cycle two or three times, pausing after each time to observe any changes.

Four-phase fascia breathing

Fascia breathing connects active and passive inhalations and exhalations. The aim is to evenly stretch the inner fascial network as much as possible (by inhaling) and then contract the respiratory fascia with an active exhalation. This creates a continuous transition between tension and compression affecting the inner respiratory network, with the same effect as physical exercise. This stretching and contracting produces a constant exchange. Tension and compression – always in transition. The tissue is squeezed like a sponge and then refills during the relief phase.

Exhalation: Active
Inhalation: Passive

You can feel how your breathing moves you, although you are seemingly sitting motionless. This is exactly the point of this exercise: deepening the feeling of elasticity in order to optimise your breathing. It's not a question of breathing forcefully or quickly. Let your breath determine the tempo.

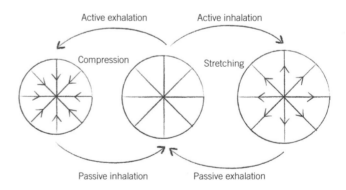

133

How it works

Come into an upright yet relaxed seated position. Become aware of your inhalations and exhalations, as well as the pauses between them, for a couple of breaths.

» Active inhaling: breathe in gently at the midpoint of your breath cycle. Feel the breath in your nostrils as it flows into and fills your body. Let your inhaling become as deep as possible, as if you wanted to expand your whole upper body - your front body, ribs, back and perhaps even your arms.
» Passive exhaling: let your breath flow out, relaxed, until you come back to the midpoint of your breath cycle.
» Active exhaling: from the midpoint, breathe out as gently as possible. The exhalation is now active. The previously stretched fascial tissue in the abdomen now becomes shorter and firmer. Active exhaling is supported by active tension in the abdomen. At the end of your exhalation, you feel like you have exhaled everything.
» Passive inhaling: let your breath start flowing back in naturally. The body finds itself back at the midpoint of the breath. Here, start actively inhaling again. The breath cycle thus continues uninterrupted.

Repeat this breath cycle for 20 to 30 breaths. Then let your breath return to a free, relaxed flow, in and out.

Final relaxation

Perhaps the most well-known relaxation pose in yoga is "corpse pose". The body lies absolutely still on the mat. At first glance, this seems like one of the easiest exercises, but accepting the stillness is sometimes more difficult than it appears. It is often much easier to be active. The aim is not only to accept the stillness of the body – it is much more important to bring stillness to the mind. In many cases, it is only when we are perfectly still and immobile that we notice how much movement and restlessness rule our thoughts, stopping the mind from relaxing. Observe your thoughts, and perhaps this exercise will show you what drives and preoccupies you internally.

How it works

» Lie on your back in a relaxed position. Place your arms to the sides of your body, with your palms facing the ceiling. The legs lie relaxed on the mat, and the feet fall outwards slightly. Close your eyes. Feel the floor under your body. Feel yourself being held, and sink further and further into your mat.

If you have practised for 60 minutes, you should spend six to eight minutes in the relaxation pose. For longer sessions, you can also plan a longer relaxation time.

Tips for relaxation

Comfortable lying position: If you find lying on your back uncomfortable, change the position of your legs. Bend your knees or lay a blanket or your fascia roller under your knees to relieve your back.

Comfortable temperature: Make sure your body doesn't cool down. Keep a jacket and warm socks ready if you tend to feel cold, because you cannot relax fully if you are cold.

Falling asleep: You may notice that you fall asleep or become dozy at the end of the relaxation. This probably means your body needs it! Next time, vary your position and observe whether you fall asleep again.

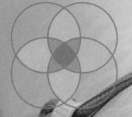

Chapter 9

Exercise sequences

How do I put together a fascia yoga session?

In the previous chapters, you have been introduced to many exercises from all five parts of fascia yoga. You've looked at each petal of the fascia yoga flower separately. The following sequences of exercises encourage you to see and experience the flower as a whole. I have put together sensible sequences of exercises for you, for different performance levels and objectives. These sessions are only recommendations. In keeping with the principles of fascia yoga, I invite you to let your own creativity guide you. With the catalogue of exercises presented here, we have laid the foundations for a modular, creative and joyful fascia yoga practice.

Let your fascia yoga flower bloom again and again. Keep adding to your yoga practice with new stimuli and new movements – you are sure to have fun doing so!

When putting together a practice, keep the following in mind:

» Before starting the exercises, take a few moments to bring your thoughts and awareness inwards and onto the mat. Close your eyes for two to three minutes and observe your breath. This time of stillness and quiet allows you to be relaxed and focused as you begin your fascia yoga.

» Wherever possible, make sure to include all five training elements (the five petals of the fascia yoga flower) in each yoga session. This ensures a truly complete fascia yoga practice.

» Practise the fascia salutation! It is fun, and a wonderful way to warm up.

» Start with gentle techniques like rolling and stretching. When your body has warmed up a little, you can also include exercises from "Strong and stable" and "Swing, bounce and jump".

» Breathing exercises are best practised at the start and/or end of your fascia yoga session.

» End each fascia yoga session with a final relaxation exercise (chapter 8). Indulge your body with quiet relaxation after a session with lots of movement.

Classic fascia salutation

The sun salutation is probably the most well-known sequence of exercises in yoga. You might have already practised one of the many variations. The classic sun salutation comprises 12 exercises, beginning and ending in mountain pose. Each movement is made in connection with the breath, giving a constant exchange between expansion (becoming taller and wider) and contraction (becoming smaller, sinking down).

The fascia salutation follows the major principles of the yoga poses in the sun salutation, but includes additional elements of fascia yoga. You stretch, bounce and jump in three dimensions. We use the exercises from the sections "Lengthen and extend", "Strong and stable" and "Swing, bounce and jump". You have already been introduced to all the exercises in previous chapters.

The fascia salutation:

» stretches the whole front and back body
» connects your breathing with the movements
» boosts the whole fascial network
» mobilises almost all the joints in the body – particularly the spine, hips and shoulders, which are important for fascia yoga
» activates the core (deep front fascial chain)
» reinvigorates and warms the body.

Let's go!

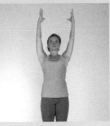

1. Inhale to mountain (see page 94)

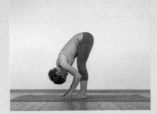

2. Exhale to standing forward fold (see page 52)

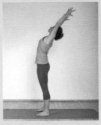

3. Inhale to rounded back, rolling into mountain with tension (see page 122)

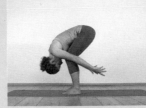

4. Exhale to swing flexibly into forward fold (see page 122)

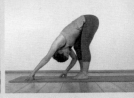

5. Two breaths, diagonal stretching (see page 52)

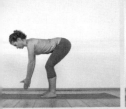

6. Inhale to straight back (see page 114)

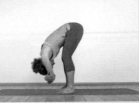

7. Exhale to pulsing forward fold (see page 109)

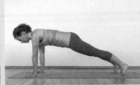

8. Inhale to high plank (see page 96)

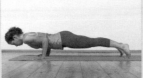

9. Exhale to low plank (see page 97)

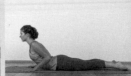

10. Inhale to cobra (see page 64)

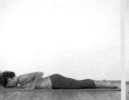

11. Exhale to lying flat on the stomach

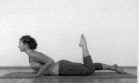

12. Inhale to bend the left knee to one-legged cobra (see page 64)

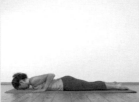

13. Exhale to lying flat on the stomach

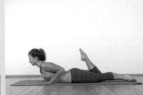

14. Inhale to bend the right knee to one-legged cobra (see page 64)

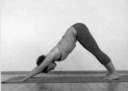

15. Exhale to downward-facing dog (see page 54)

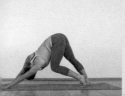

16. Two breaths in lolling dog (see page 54)

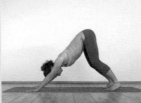

17. Inhale to dancing dog with pulsing heels (see page 107)

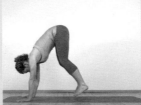

18. Exhale to springing dog into forward fold (see page 117)

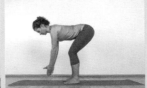

19. Inhale to straight back (see page 114)

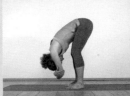

20. Exhale to pulsing forward fold (see page 109)

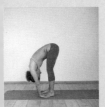

21. Inhale to pulsing upright (see page 123)

The fascia salutation

Classic fascia salutation plus

Expand the classic fascia salutation with powerful dynamic elements that you have already seen in the sections "Lengthen and extend" and "Swing, bounce and jump". Moving from downward-facing dog (see page 139, fig. 15), move one leg forward into high lunge. From here, you can include various warrior and triangle variations, bringing even more elastic elements (swinging warrior and springing dog) into the fascia salutation.

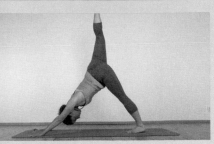

16. Inhale to three-legged dog (lifting the right leg, see page 83)

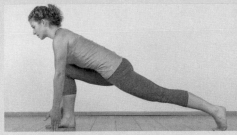

17. Exhale to high lunge (see page 26)

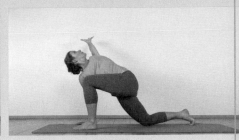

18. Inhale to revolved side angle, variation 1 with wide opening (see page 84)

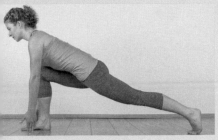

19. Exhale to high lunge (see page 26)

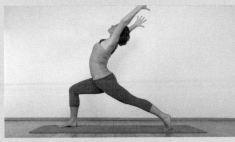

20. Inhale to warrior (see page 62)

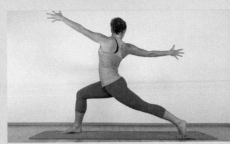

21. Two to three breaths in fighting warrior (see page 63)

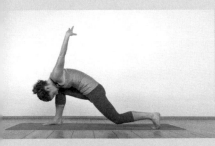

22. Exhale to swinging warrior into high lunge (see page 124)

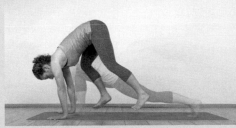

23. Inhale to jumping lunge (see page 120). Repeat on the left side from high lunge (17) to swinging warrior (22)

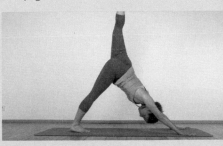

24. Inhale to three-legged dog (lifting the left leg, see page 83)

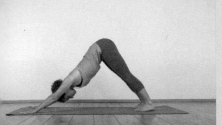

25. Exhale to downward-facing dog (see page 54)

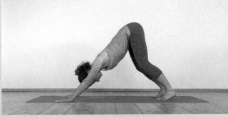

26. Inhale to dancing dog with pulsing heels (see page 107)

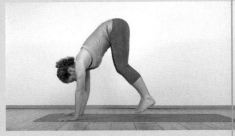

27. Exhale to springing dog into forward fold (see page 117)

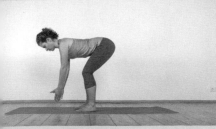

28. Inhale to straight back (see page 114)

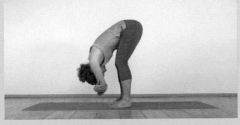

29. Exhale to pulsing forward fold (see page 109)

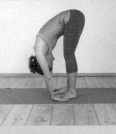

30. Inhale to pulsing upright (see page 123)

Easy fascia salutation

This easy variation is a good introduction, not only for novice yogis but also for any who want to gently prepare their fascia for the classic fascia salutation. The focus here is on the stretches. We remove the stronger elements like high plank and low plank. You come to the ground from tabletop position and replace cobra with cow. The swinging elements are also replaced with fascial stretching.

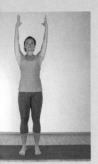

1. Inhale to mountain
(see page 94)

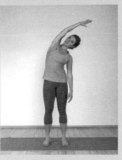

2. Two breaths in palm in
the wind (see page 108)

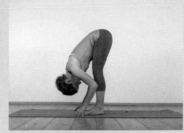

3. Exhale to standing forward fold
(see page 52)

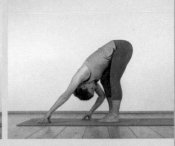

4. Two breaths in diagonal
stretching (see page 142)

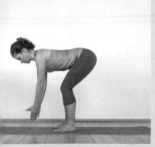

5. Inhale to straight back
(see page 114)

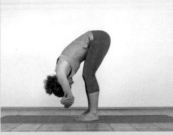

6. Exhale to pulsing forward fold
(see page 109)

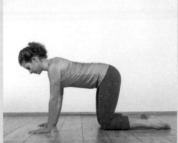

7. Inhale to tabletop position
(see page 26)

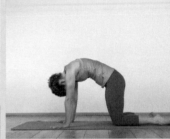

8. Exhale to cat (see page 60)

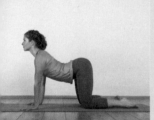

9. Inhale to cow (see page 69)

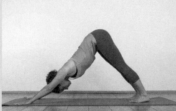

10. Exhale to downward-facing dog
(see page 54)

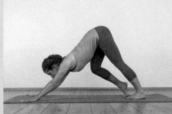

11. Two breaths in lolling dog
(see page 54)

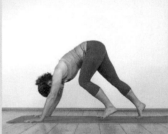

12. Inhale to smoothly walk up
to your hands

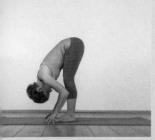

13. Exhale to standing
forward fold (see page 52)

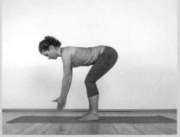

14. Inhale to straight back
(see page 114)

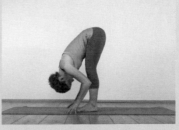

15. Exhale to standing forward fold
(see page 52)

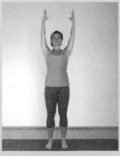

16. Inhale to mountain
(see page 94)

Fascia yoga for beginners

This sequence is a good introduction to fascia yoga. I have put together the easiest exercises from each section for you, so that you can start without any prior knowledge of yoga. The unit is designed to reach all fascial chains to a balanced degree. Give yourself time to practise and only go as far as is comfortable for you.

Arriving: Take two to three minutes to arrive on your mat. Close your eyes and concentrate on your breathing and on maintaining an upright sitting position.

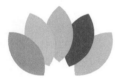

Breathing

Begin the session with a breathing exercise. You will notice that these first few minutes during which you focus all your awareness on yourself bring calm. Your breathing becomes more conscious, the breaths a little deeper, and your fascia yoga session more intense and effective.

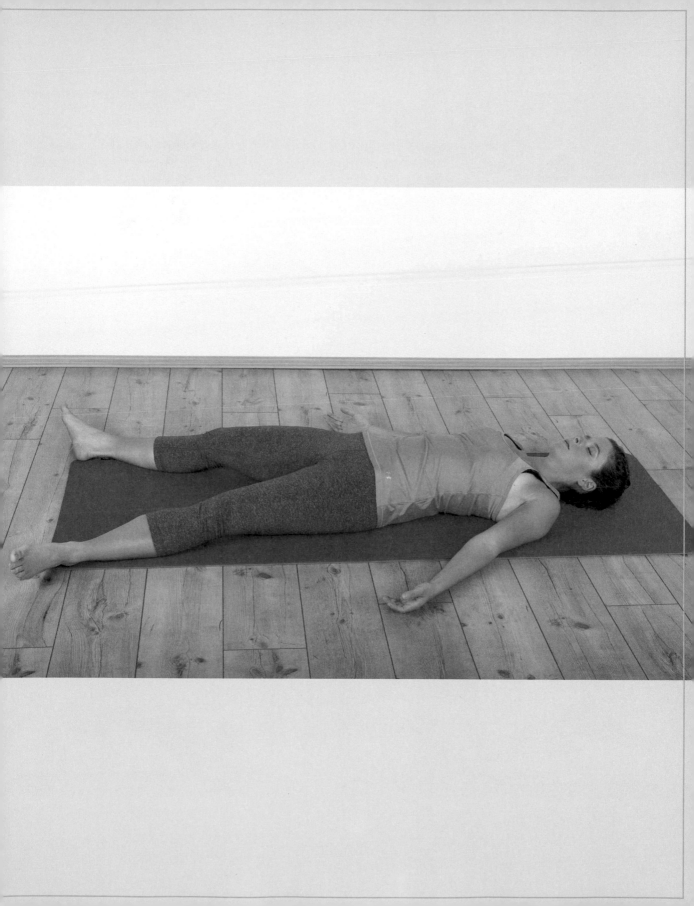

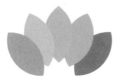

Releasing tension

Self-massage with a fascia roller and fascia balls is a wonderful start to a fascia yoga practice. This rolling stimulates the blood flow to the muscle and fascial tissues and gently releases tensions and even painful stuck areas. I have already presented the basic principles in chapter 4. Rolling selected parts of the body is the perfect way to prepare the body for various yoga exercises, so that they become even more intense and beneficial.

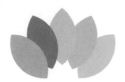

Strong and stable: Flow 1

This short flow strengthens your posture and upright position. Breathe more length into your body with each inhalation, and stabilise this length as you exhale. This flow becomes dynamic thanks to the association of breath and movement. You may even feel a little taller afterwards!

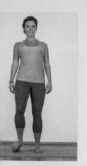

1. Soles of the feet
(see page 31)

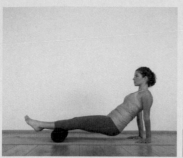

2. Calves (see page 34)

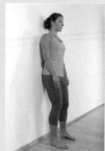

3. Hamstrings (see page 37)

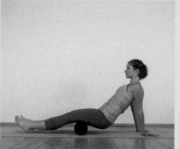

4. Outer thighs (see page 38)

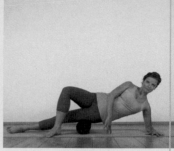

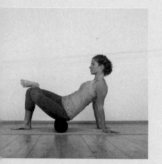

5. Buttocks with roller
(see page 40)

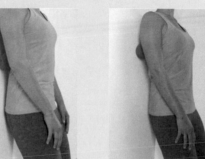

6–8. Standing back massage (lower back, thoracic spine and shoulder with ball,
see page 44)

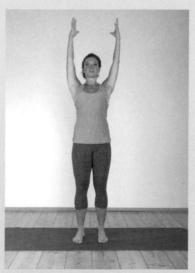

1. Inhale to mountain (see page 94)

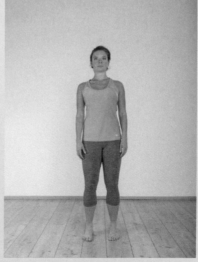

2. Exhale to standing upright (see
page 23). Repeat for ten breaths

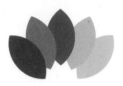

Easy fascia salutation

This easy variation is a good introduction, not only for novice yogis but also for any who want to gently prepare their fascia for the classic fascia salutation. The focus here is on the stretches. We remove the stronger elements like high plank and low plank. You come to the ground from tabletop position and replace cobra with cow. The swinging elements are also replaced with fascial stretching.

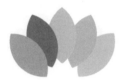

Strong and stable: Flow 2

Another short flow to boost your whole body. The dynamic changing from mountain to lightning bolt produces a fair amount of heat, as this combination of movements incorporates the majority of your muscles.

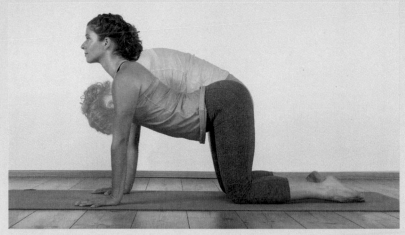

Easy fascia salutation (see pages 142–43)

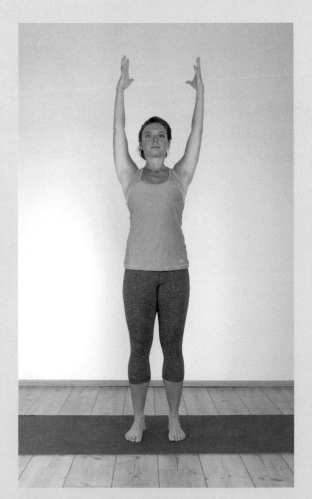

1. Inhale to mountain (see page 94)

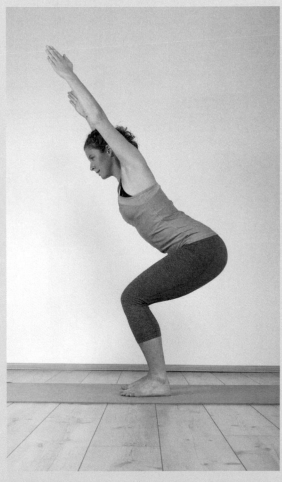

2. Exhale to lightning bolt (see page 95). Repeat for ten breaths

**Special
sequences for
beginners**

Lengthen and extend

Our fascia loves to be stretched out. With these carefully selected exercises, you can reach all the fascial chains that run through the body. Stay active in the poses, either by constantly changing the tensile load or by including small, gentle swinging movements. After these exercises, your body will feel much more supple and mobile.

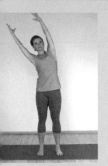
1. Standing crescent
(see page 72)

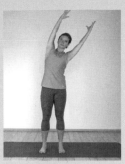
2. Changing moon
(see page 72)

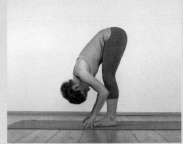
3. Standing forward fold
(see page 52)

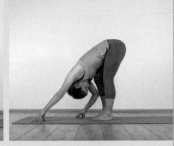
4. Diagonal stretching
(see page 52)

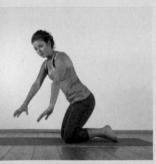
5. Cat (see page 60)

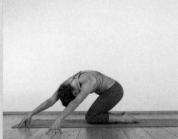
6. Cow (see page 69)

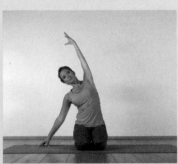
7. Ten breaths, alternating cat–cow

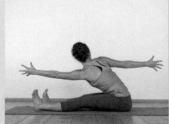
8. Wild cat (see page 60)

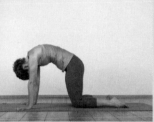
9. Springing cat
(see page 116)

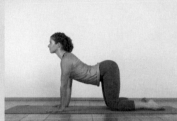
10. Moving child (see page 59)

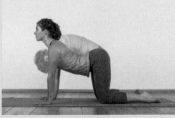
11. Side arch (see page 74)

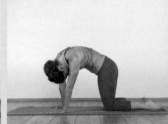
12. Seated forward fold with
stretching (see page 53)

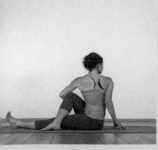
13. Sitting half spinal twist
(see page 87)

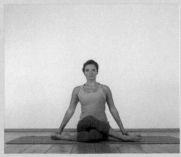
14. Shoelace (see page 73)

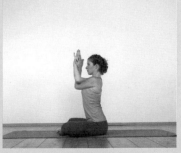
15. Eagle arms (see page 89)

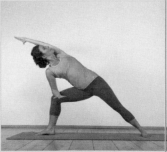
16. Extended side angle
(see page 77)

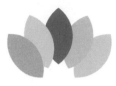

Swing, bounce and jump

Now it's time to be dynamic. The exercises selected bring elasticity to your fascial network. Energetic swinging, loose pulsing and lively springing movements promote collagen synthesis in the fascial tissue and ensure firm but flexible fascia. Here, I have collected gentle exercises that incorporate all the major fascial chains.

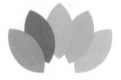

Strong and stable

The core is key to our posture and movements. The deep fascial chain acts as our internal stabiliser. Without it, our posture would be unstable and our movements weak. In addition to the dynamic flows, I also recommend a standing pose that encourages you to ground into the mat and align your posture.

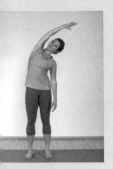

1. Palm in the wind
(see page 108)

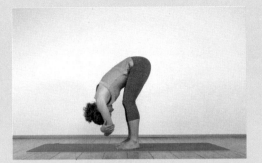

2. Pulsing forward fold (see page 109)

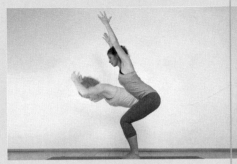

3. Lightning bolt and forward fold
(see page 110)

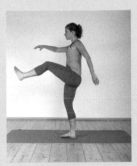

4. Leg swing (see page 112)

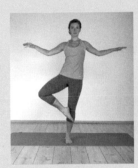

5. Figure of eight
(see page 113)

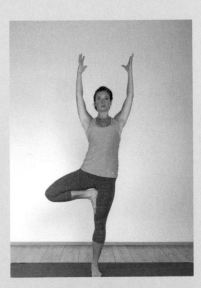

1. Tree (see page 101)

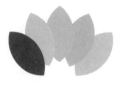

Relaxing stretches

After tensing, don't forget to relax at the end of your session. The relaxing stretches at the end of a session release and harmonise the structures you have been working. Take at least ten breaths, or even longer, to stay in the poses.

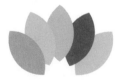

Final relaxation

Take five to ten minutes at the end of each session to relax in corpse pose, in order to allow your body, breathing and mind to come back to a calm state after the practice. Relaxing at the end of the session is a beneficial source of energy for your body.

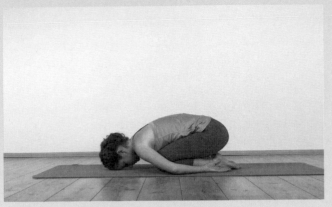
1. Child (see page 59)

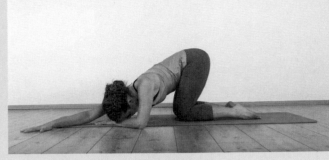
2. Sideways child (see page 78)

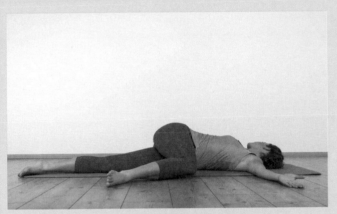
3. Knee down twist (see page 86)

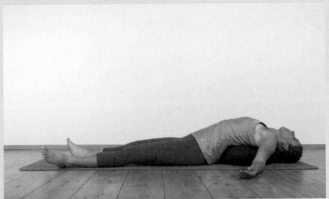
4. Fish using a meditation cushion (see page 70)

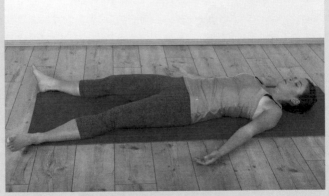
1. Final relaxation (see page 134)

Fascia yoga for experienced yogis

This sequence brings together all the elements of fascia yoga. The movement flows put together here are strong and dynamic, while the stretches are demanding yet soothing. Take the time to experiment and enjoy the sensations.

Arriving: Take two to three minutes to arrive on your mat. Close your eyes and concentrate on your breathing and maintaining an upright sitting position.

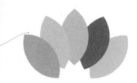

Breathing

Begin the session with a breathing exercise. You will notice that these first few minutes during which you focus all your awareness on yourself bring calm. Your breathing becomes more conscious, the breaths a little deeper, and your fascia yoga session more intense and effective.

Releasing tension

Self-massage with a fascia roller and fascia balls is a wonderful start to a fascia yoga practice. This rolling stimulates the blood flow to the muscle and fascial tissues and gently releases tensions and even painful stuck areas. I have already presented the basic principles in chapter 4. Rolling selected parts of the body is the perfect way to prepare the body for various yoga exercises, so that they become even more intense and beneficial.

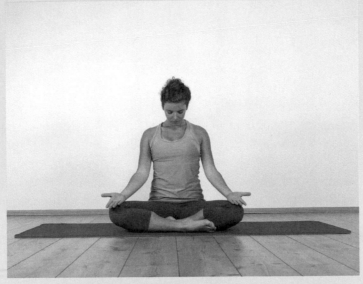

1. Fascia breathing (see page 133). Kapalabhati (see page 131)

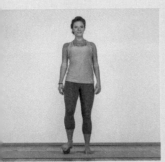

1. Soles of the feet (see page 31)

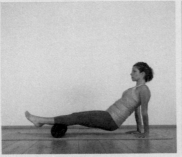

2. Calves (see page 34)

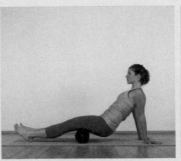

3. Hamstrings (see page 37)

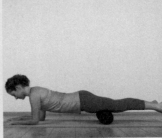

4. Thighs (see page 36)

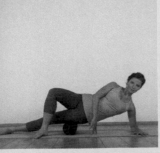

5. Outer thighs (see page 38)

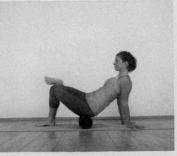

6. Buttocks with roller (see page 40)

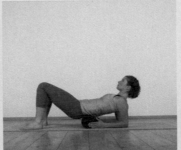

7. Lower back (see page 41)

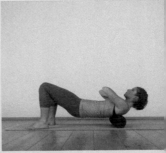

8. Upper back (see page 43)

**Special sequences
for experienced
yogis**

Classic fascia salutation

The fascia salutation follows the major principles of the yoga poses in the sun salutation, but includes additional elements of fascia yoga. You stretch, bounce and jump in three dimensions. We use the exercises from the sections "Lengthen and extend", "Strong and stable" and "Swing, bounce and jump". You have already been introduced to all the exercises in previous chapters.

Classic fascia salutation plus

Expand the classic fascia salutation with powerful dynamic elements that you have already seen in the sections "Lengthen and extend" and "Swing, bounce and jump". Moving from downward-facing dog, move one leg forward into high lunge. From here, you can include various warrior and triangle variations, bringing even more elastic elements (swinging warrior and springing dog) into the fascia salutation.

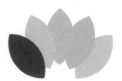

Lengthen and extend

Our fascia loves to be stretched out. With these carefully selected exercises, you can reach all the fascial chains that run through the body. Stay active in the poses, either by constantly changing the tensile load or by including small, gentle swinging movements. After these exercises, your body will feel much more supple and mobile.

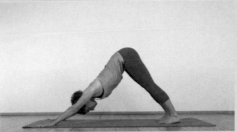

Classic fascia salutation (see pages 138–39); repeat four times

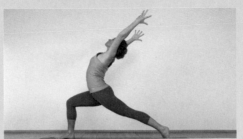

Fascia salutation plus (see pages 140–41); repeat twice

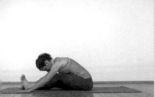

1. Extending the back fascial chain (see page 53)

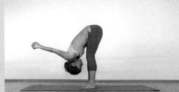

2. Forward fold with pulsing arms (see page 91)

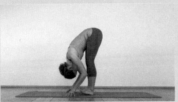

3. Forward fold with transfer of weight (see page 52)

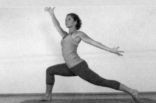

4. Fighting warrior (see page 63)

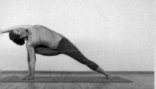

5. Extended side angle (see page 77)

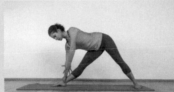

6. Circling triangle (see page 76)

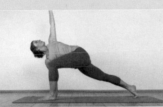

7. Revolved side angle with opening (see page 81)

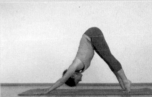

8. Big dog (see page 54)

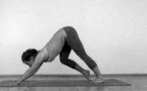

9. Lolling dog (see page 54)

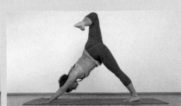

10. Three-legged dog with twist (see page 83)

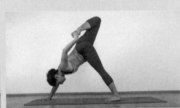

11. Two-legged dog (see page 83)

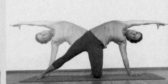

12. Gate (see page 75)

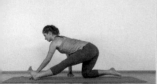

13. Half pyramid with exploring (see page 58)

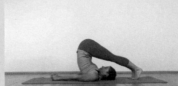

14. Plow (see page 56)

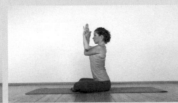

15. Eagle arms (see page 89)

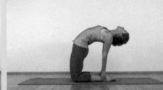

16. Camel/one-armed camel (see page 67)

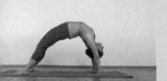

17. Wheel (see page 66)

**Special sequences
for experienced
yogis**

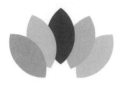

Swing, bounce and jump

Now it's time to be dynamic. The exercises selected bring elasticity to your fascial network. Energetic swinging, loose pulsing and lively springing movements promote collagen synthesis in the fascial tissue and ensure firm but flexible fascia.

The exercises selected reach all the long fascial chains in your body and will boost your circulation.

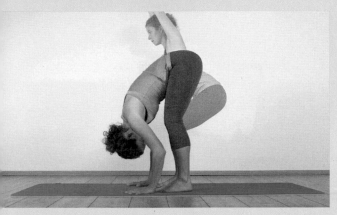

1. Lightning bolt and forward fold (see page 110)

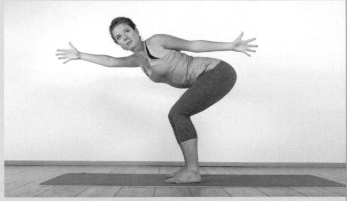

2. Flat back with swinging arms (see page 114)

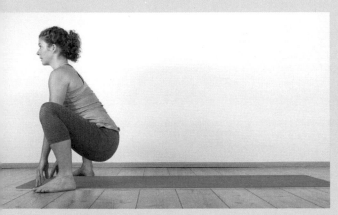

3. Frog jump (see page 119)

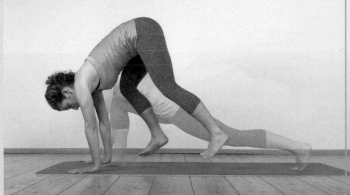

4. Jumping lunge (see page 120)

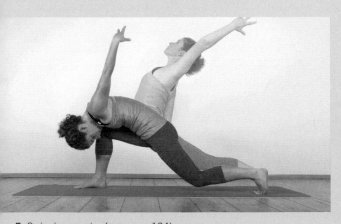

5. Swinging warrior (see page 124)

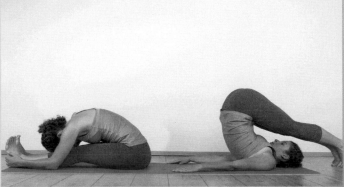

6. Plow and rolling (see page 125)

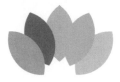

**Special sequences
for experienced
yogis**

Strong and stable

The core is key to our posture and movements. The deep fascial chain acts as our internal stabiliser. Without it, our posture would be unstable and our movements weak. I have put together a short but very intense flow for you that reaches the core and requires strength in the arms and shoulders.

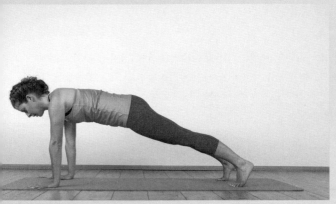

1. Exhale to high plank (see page 96)

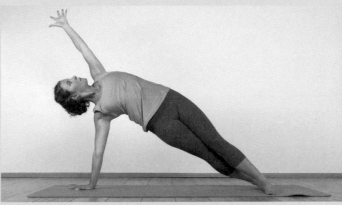

2. Inhale to side plank on right, hold for two breaths (see page 98)

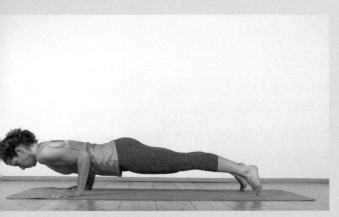

3. Exhale to low plank (see page 97)

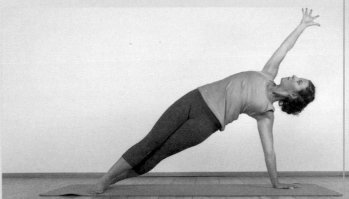

4. Inhale to side plank on left, hold for two breaths (see page 98)

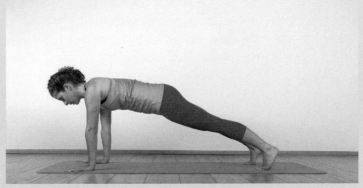

5. Exhale to high plank (see page 96)

Special sequences for experienced yogis

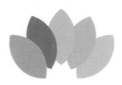

Additions for the core

Add to this flow with poses that again strengthen the core in a targeted way (boat, half boat and windscreen wipers). Hold them for five to ten breaths. Practice makes perfect. You will notice that you can gradually increase the number of breaths, or repeat the exercises two or three times.

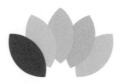

Relaxing stretches

After tensing, don't forget to relax at the end of your session. The relaxing stretches at the end of a session release and harmonise the structures you have been working. Take at least ten breaths, or even longer, to stay in the poses.

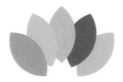

Final relaxation

Take five to ten minutes at the end of each session to relax in corpse pose, in order to allow your body, breathing and mind to come back to a calm state after the practice. Relaxing at the end of the session is a beneficial source of energy for your body.

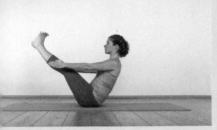

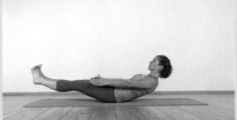

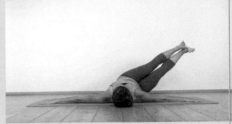

1. Boat (see page 99)

2. Half boat (see page 99)

3. Windscreen wipers (see page 100)

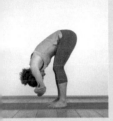

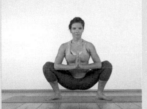

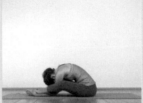

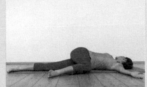

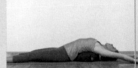

1. Pulsing forward fold (see page 109)

2. Garland (see page 103)

3. Tortoise (see page 102)

4. Knee down twist (see page 86)

5. Fish using a meditation cushion (see page 70)

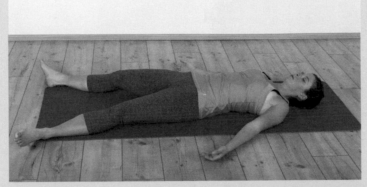

1. Final relaxation (see page 134)

Fascia yoga for relaxation

Sometimes, it is not easy to just relax, as our daily lives are often full of rushing around and deadlines. But it is important to take breaks and recharge your batteries. In the following sequence, I've collected together relaxing and particularly soothing exercises for you. Here, we focus on fascial stretches and exercises that allow the body to hang loosely and swing freely. Rolling is included at the end of the session, so that you can gently stretch any tight areas and then sink fully relaxed into the stillness.

Breathing

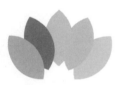

Begin the session with a breathing exercise. You will notice that these first few minutes during which you focus all your awareness on yourself bring calm. Your breathing becomes more conscious, the breaths a little deeper, and your fascia yoga session more intense and effective.

Strong and stable

The core is key to our posture and movements. The deep fascial chain acts as our internal stabiliser. Without it, our posture would be unstable and our movements weak. This short flow strengthens your posture and upright position. Breathe more length into your body with each inhalation, and stabilise this length as you exhale. This flow becomes dynamic thanks to the association of breath and movement. You may even feel a little taller afterwards! Plank strengthens your whole body and is a great all-rounder for reinforcing your core.

Easy fascia salutation

This easy variation is a good introduction, not only for novice yogis but also for any who want to gently prepare their fascia for the classic fascia salutation. The focus here is on the stretches. We remove the stronger elements like high plank and low plank. You come to the ground from tabletop position and replace cobra with cow. The swinging elements are also replaced with fascial stretching.

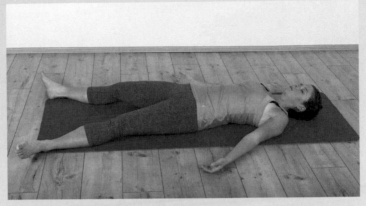

Full yoga breathing (see page 131). Fascia breathing (see page 133)

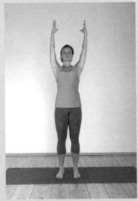

1. Inhale to mountain (see page 94)

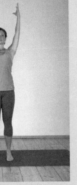

2. Exhale to standing position (see page 23). Repeat for ten breaths

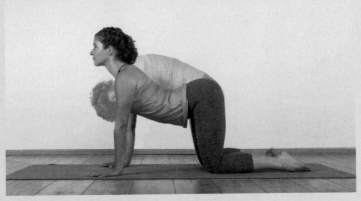

Easy fascia salutation (see page 142); repeat four to six times

**Special sequences
for relaxing**

Lengthen and extend

Our fascia loves to be stretched out. With these carefully selected exercises, you can reach all the fascial chains that run through the body. Stay active in the poses, either by constantly changing the tensile load or by including small, gentle swinging movements. After these exercises, your body will feel much more supple and mobile.

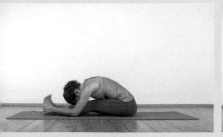

1. Seated forward fold (see page 53)

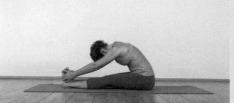

2. Rounded back (see page 53)

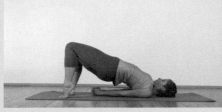

3. Pelvic swing (see page 66)

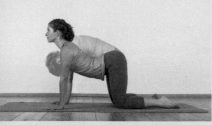

4. Cat–cow (inhale to cow, exhale to cat; see pages 60 and 69)

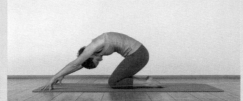

5. Moving child (see page 59)

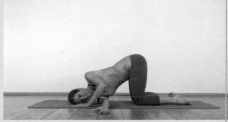

6. Thread the needle (see page 84)

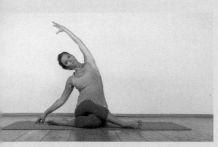

7. Shoelace with side bend (see page 73)

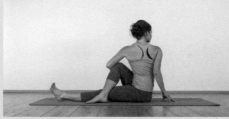

8. Sitting half spinal twist (see page 87)

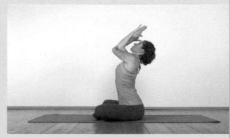

9. Flying eagle (see page 89)

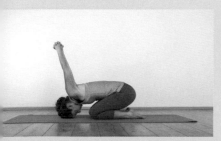

10. Child with clasped hands (see page 91)

**Special sequences
for relaxing**

Swing, bounce and jump

Now it's time to be dynamic. The exercises selected bring elasticity to your fascial network. Energetic swinging, loose pulsing and lively springing movements promote collagen synthesis in the fascial tissue and ensure firm but flexible fascia.

The exercises selected are loose swinging movements, in which the spine can completely "let go". The shoulders and neck are also loosened.

Relaxing stretches

After tensing, don't forget to relax at the end of your session. The relaxing stretches at the end of a session release and harmonise the structures you have been working. Take at least ten breaths, or even longer, to stay in the poses.

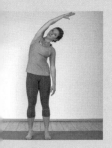

1. Palm in the wind
(see page 108)

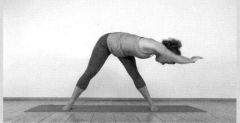

2. Standing straight angle pose with swinging upper body (see page 111)

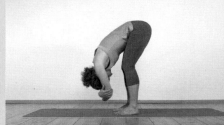

3. Pulsing forward fold (see page 109)

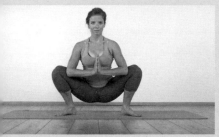

1. Garland (see page 103)

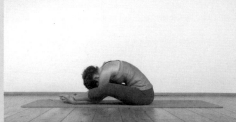

2. Tortoise (see page 102)

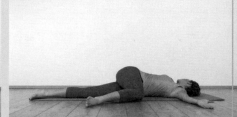

3. Knee down twist (see page 86)

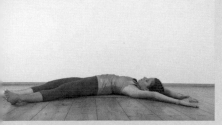

4. Lying crescent (see page 79)

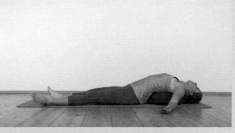

5. Fish using a meditation cushion
(see page 70)

Special sequences for relaxing

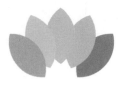

Releasing tension

Self-massage with a fascia roller and fascia balls can also be a wonderful way to end your fascia yoga session. Rolling gently loosens tense or even painful stuck areas. I have already presented the basic principles in chapter 4. By rolling specific parts of your body, you reduce the level of tension in the muscle and encourage the body to regenerate and relax.

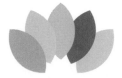

Final relaxation

Take five to ten minutes at the end of each session to relax in corpse pose, in order to allow your body, breathing and mind to come back to a calm state after the practice. Relaxing at the end of the session is a beneficial source of energy for your body.

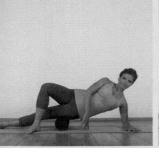 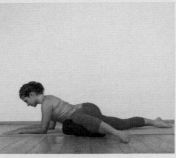 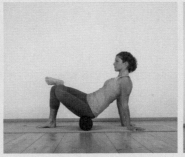 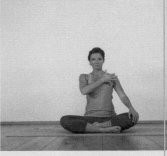

1. Outer thighs (see page 38)   **2.** Inner thighs (see page 39)   **3.** Buttocks with roller (see page 40)   **4.** Chest muscles (see page 45)

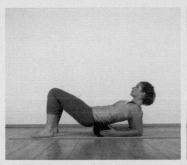 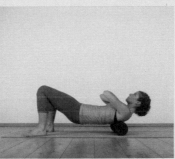 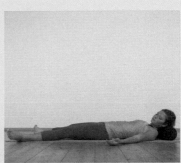

5. Lower back (see page 41)   **6.** Upper back (see page 43)   **7.** Neck (see page 46)

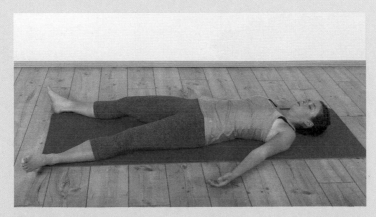

Final relaxation (see page 134)

Fascia yoga for a healthy back

Some of the most commonly encountered physical complaints are tension and pain in the back and shoulders/neck. And it's no wonder – we generally move less than our bodies need. The following sequence strengthens your whole back, and mobilises your hips, shoulders and spine. Shortened parts are lengthened again. The swinging exercises return movement and elasticity to your large back fascia.

Arriving: Take two to three minutes to arrive on your mat. Close your eyes and concentrate on your breathing and on maintaining an upright sitting position.

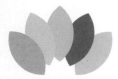

Breathing

Begin the session with a breathing exercise. You will notice that these first few minutes during which you focus all your awareness on yourself bring calm. Your breathing becomes more conscious, the breaths a little deeper, and your fascia yoga session more intense and effective.

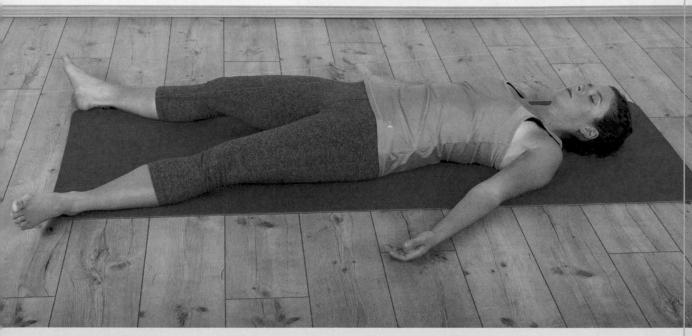

Full yoga breathing (see page 131)
Fascia breathing (see page 133)

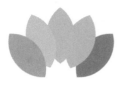

Releasing tension

Self-massage with a fascia roller and fascia balls is a wonderful start to a fascia yoga practice. This rolling stimulates the blood flow to the muscle and fascial tissues and gently releases tensions and even painful stuck areas. I have already presented the basic principles in chapter 4. Rolling selected parts of the body is the perfect way to prepare the body for various yoga exercises, so that they become even more intense and beneficial.

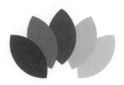

Easy fascia salutation

This easy variation is a good introduction, not only for novice yogis but also for any who want to gently prepare their fascia for the classic fascia salutation. The focus here is on the stretches. We remove the stronger elements like high plank and low plank. You come to the ground from tabletop position and replace cobra with cow. The swinging elements are also replaced with fascial stretching.

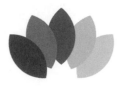

Classic fascia salutation

The fascia salutation follows the major principles of the yoga poses in the sun salutation, but includes additional elements of fascia yoga. You stretch, bounce and jump in three dimensions. We use the exercises from the sections "Lengthen and extend", "Strong and stable" and "Swing, bounce and jump". You have already been introduced to all the exercises in previous chapters.

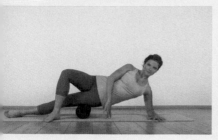

1. Outer thighs (see page 38)

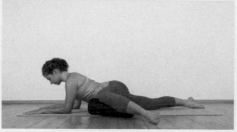

2. Inner thighs (see page 39)

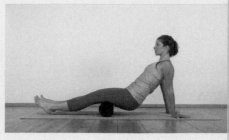

3. Hamstrings (see page 37)

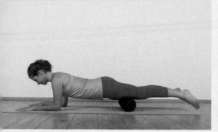

4. Thighs (see page 36)

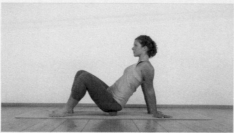

5. Buttocks with roller and/or ball (see page 40)

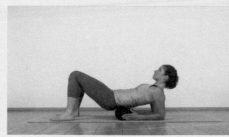

6. Lower back (see page 41)

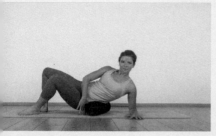

7. Side body (see page 42)

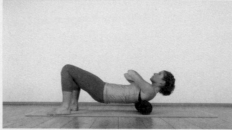

8. Upper back (see page 43)

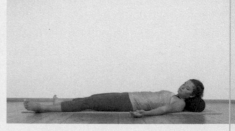

9. Neck (see page 46)

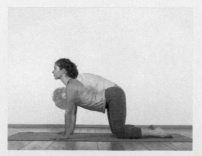

Easy fascia salutation (see pages 142–43);
repeat four to six times

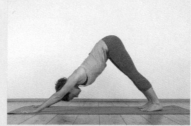

Classic fascia salutation (see pages 138–39);
repeat twice

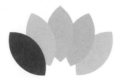

**Special
sequences for
the back**

Lengthen and extend

Our fascia loves to be stretched out. With these carefully selected exercises, you can reach all the fascial chains that run through the body. Stay active in the poses, either by constantly changing the tensile load or by including small, gentle swinging movements. After these exercises, your body will feel much more supple and mobile.

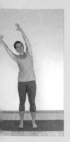

1. Standing crescent
(see page 72)

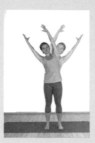

2. Changing moon (see page 72)

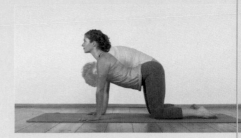

3. Cat–cow (inhale to cow, exhale to cat;
see pages 60 and 69)

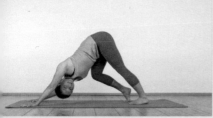

4. Wild cat (see page 60)

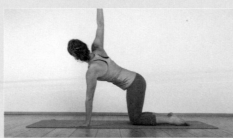

5. "Up and down" threading (see page 84)

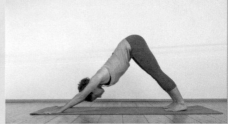

6. Downward-facing dog (see page 54)

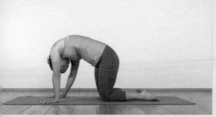

7. Lolling dog (see page 54)

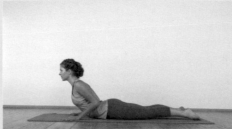

8. Cobra (see page 64)

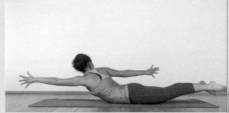

9. Curious cobra (see page 65)

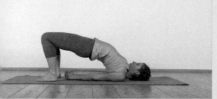

10. Bridge (inhale to lift, exhale
to come back down; see page 66)

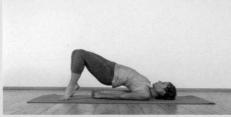

11. Pelvic swing (see page 66)

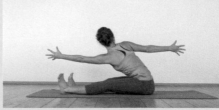

12. Seated forward fold with diagonal
stretching (see page 53)

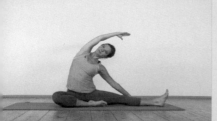

13. "Up and down" gate (see page 75)

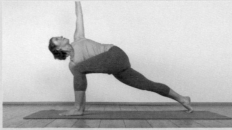

14. Revolved side angle (see page 81)

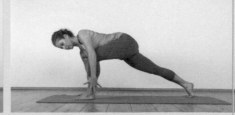

15. Circling angle (see page 82)

Special
sequences for
the back

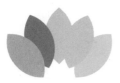

Strong and stable

The core is key to our posture and movements. The deep fascial chain acts as our internal stabiliser. Without it, our posture would be unstable and our movements weak. This short flow strengthens your posture and upright position, and reaches nearly every part of the body.

Additions for the core

Add to this flow with poses that again strengthen the core in a targeted way (side plank, boat and windscreen wipers). Hold them for five to ten breaths. Practice makes perfect. You will notice that you can gradually increase the number of breaths, or repeat the exercises two or three times.

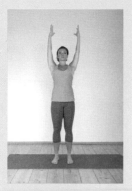

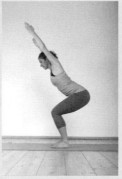

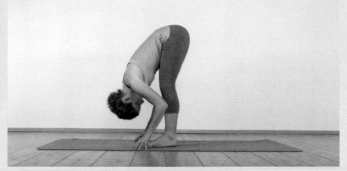

1. Inhale to mountain (see page 94)

2. Exhale and inhale in lightning bolt (see page 95)

3. Exhale to standing forward fold (see page 52)

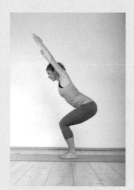

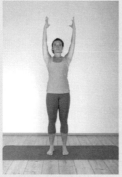

4. Exhale and inhale in lightning bolt (see page 95)

5. Inhale to mountain (see page 94)

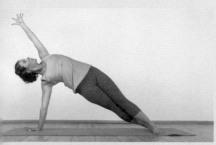

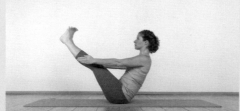

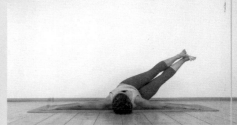

1. Side plank (see page 98)

2. Boat (see page 99)

3. Windscreen wipers (see page 100)

Special sequences for the back

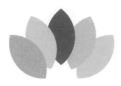

Swing, bounce and jump

Now it's time to be dynamic. The exercises selected bring elasticity to your fascial network. Energetic swinging, loose pulsing and lively springing movements promote collagen synthesis in the fascial tissue and ensure firm but flexible fascia.

The exercises selected are loose swinging movements, in which the spine can completely "let go". The shoulders and neck are also loosened.

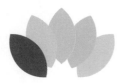

Relaxing stretches

After tensing, don't forget to relax at the end of your session. The relaxing stretches at the end of a session release and harmonise the structures you have been working. Take at least ten breaths, or even longer, to stay in the poses.

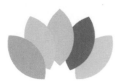

Final relaxation

Take five to ten minutes at the end of each session to relax in corpse pose, in order to allow your body, breathing and mind to come back to a calm state after the practice. Relaxing at the end of the session is a beneficial source of energy for your body.

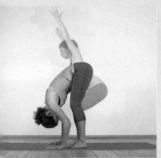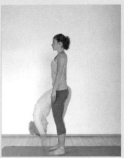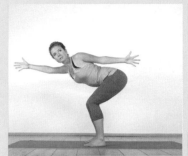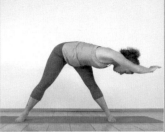

1. From mountain to forward fold (see page 122)

2. Forward fold, pulsing upright (see page 123)

3. Flat back with swinging arms (see page 114)

4. Standing straight angle pose with swinging upper body (see page 111)

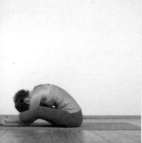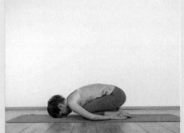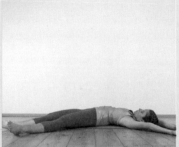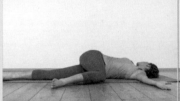

1. Tortoise (see page 102)

2. Child (see page 59)

3. Lying crescent (see page 79)

4. Knee down twist (see page 86)

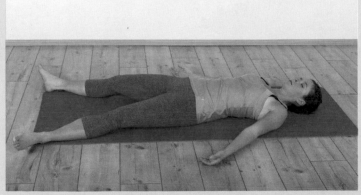

Final relaxation (see page 134)

Fascia yoga for sedentary lifestyles

Our body is not designed to sit for long periods of time, yet our daily lives mean that we are sitting for longer and longer. We typically sit at desks throughout the working day, then in a car or train on the way home, and spend our evenings sitting on the sofa. It is difficult for our bodies to cope with so little movement. When we sit, the backs of our legs are shortened while the upper part of our back is constantly stretched. Lots of sitting also shortens our front bodies. The important balance between the front and back of the body is lost over time, changing the way forces affect our whole body.

With this fascia yoga sequence, you recover this balance and bring length back into your body. Here, we focus on standing exercises and fascia stretches that reach the backs of the legs and the front body. Furthermore, your spine is gently moved in all directions and your body is woken up with inversions like downward-facing dog. The sequence is completed with dynamic exercises that being pre-tension to your front body.

Arriving: Take two to three minutes to arrive on your mat. Close your eyes and concentrate on your breathing and on maintaining an upright sitting position.

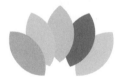

Breathing

Begin the session with a breathing exercise. You will notice that these first few minutes during which you focus all your awareness on yourself bring calm. Your breathing becomes more conscious, the breaths a little deeper, and your fascia yoga session more intense and effective.

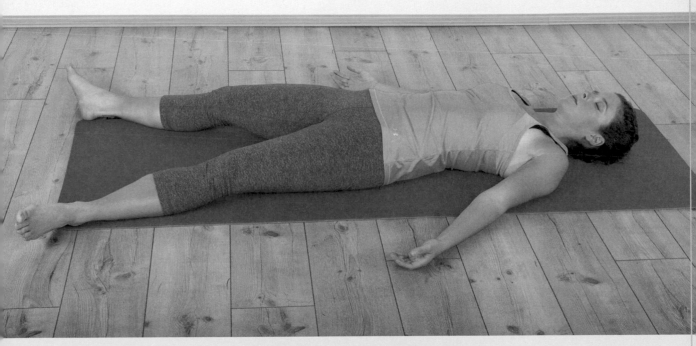

Full yoga breathing (see page 131). Kapalabhati (see page 131)

Special sequences for sedentary lifestyles

Releasing tension

Self-massage with a fascia roller and fascia balls is a wonderful start to a fascia yoga practice. This rolling stimulates the blood flow to the muscle and fascial tissues and gently releases tensions and even painful stuck areas. I have already presented the basic principles in chapter 4. Rolling selected parts of the body is the perfect way to prepare the body for various yoga exercises, so that they become even more intense and beneficial.

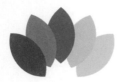

Easy fascia salutation

This easy variation is a good introduction, not only for novice yogis but also for any who want to gently prepare their fascia for the classic fascia salutation. The focus here is on the stretches. We remove the stronger elements like high plank and low plank. You come to the ground from tabletop position and replace cobra with cow. The swinging elements are also replaced with fascial stretching.

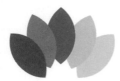

Classic fascia salutation

The fascia salutation follows the major principles of the yoga poses in the sun salutation, but includes additional elements of fascia yoga. You stretch, bounce and jump in three dimensions. We use the exercises from the sections "Lengthen and extend", "Strong and stable" and "Swing, bounce and jump". You have already been introduced to all the exercises in previous chapters.

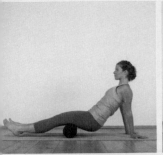

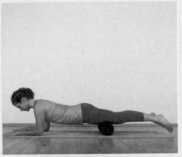

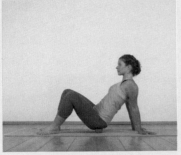

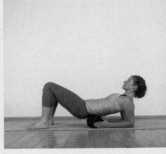

1. Hamstrings (see page 37)   **2.** Thighs (see page 36)   **3.** Buttocks with roller and/or ball (see page 40)   **4.** Lower back (see page 41)

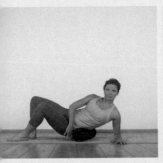

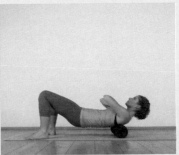

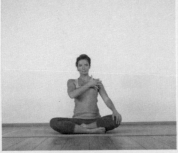

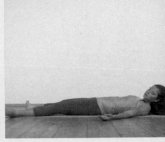

5. Side body (see page 42)   **6.** Upper back (see page 43)   **7.** Chest muscles (see page 45)   **8.** Neck (see page 46)

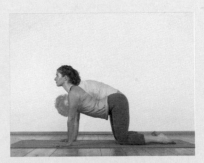

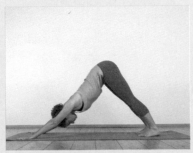

Easy fascia salutation (see pages 142–43); repeat four to six times

Classic fascia salutation (see pages 138–39); repeat twice

Special
sequences for
sedentary
lifestyles

Strong and stable

The core is key to our posture and movements. The deep fascial chain acts as our internal stabiliser. Without it, our posture would be unstable and our movements weak. This dynamic flow supports our upright posture and also strengthens the leg and shoulder muscles, often weakened by sitting.

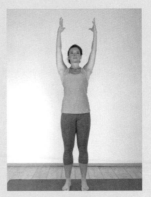
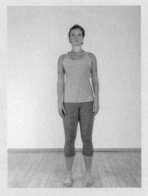
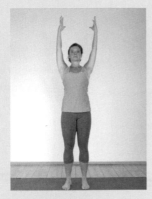

1. Inhale to mountain
(see page 94)

2. Exhale to standing position
(see page 23).
Repeat four to six times

3. Inhale to mountain
(see page 94)

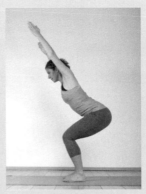
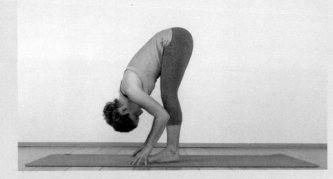

4. Exhale and inhale in
lightning bolt (see page 95)

5. Exhale to standing forward fold (see page 52)

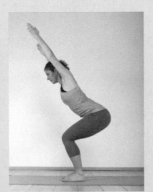
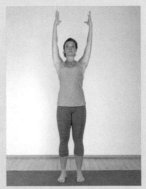

6. Exhale and inhale in
lightning bolt (see page 95)

7. Inhale to mountain
(see page 94).
Repeat four to six times

Special sequences for sedentary lifestyles

Lengthen and extend

Our fascia loves to be stretched out. With these carefully selected exercises, you can reach all the fascial chains that run through the body. Stay active in the poses, either by constantly changing the tensile load or by including small, gentle swinging movements. After these exercises, your body will feel much more supple and mobile.

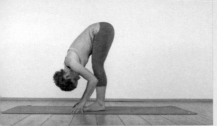 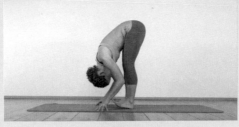 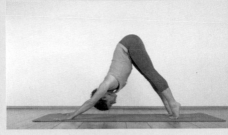

1. Standing forward fold (see page 52)

2. Forward fold with transfer of weight (see page 52)

3. Big dog (see page 54)

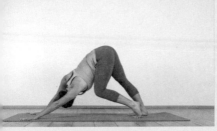 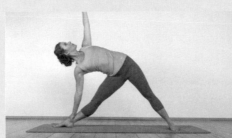 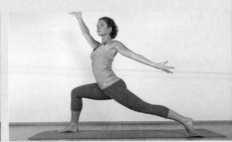

4. Lolling dog (see page 54)

5. Warrior (see page 62)

6. Fighting warrior (see page 63)

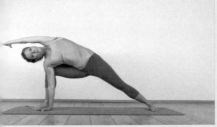 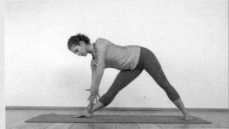

7. Extended side angle (see page 77)

8. Triangle (see page 76)

9. Circling triangle (see page 76)

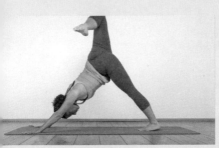 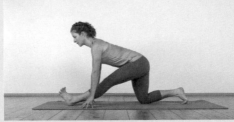 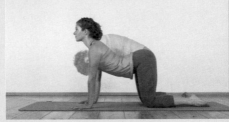

10. Three-legged dog with twist (see page 83)

11. Half pyramid (see page 58)

12. Cat–cow (inhale to cow, exhale to cat; see pages 60 and 69)

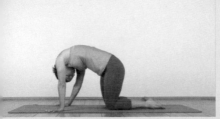 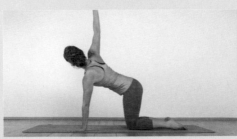

13. Wild cat (see page 60)

14. "Up and down" threading (see page 84)

Special sequences for sedentary lifestyles

Swing, bounce and jump

Now it's time to be dynamic. The exercises selected bring elasticity to your fascial network. Energetic swinging, loose pulsing and lively springing movements promote collagen synthesis in the fascial tissue and ensure firm but flexible fascia.

The exercises selected focus on the fascia in the legs, which becomes inflexible from sitting.

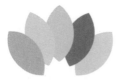

Final relaxation

Take five to ten minutes at the end of each session to relax in corpse pose, in order to allow your body, breathing and mind to come back to a calm state after the practice. Relaxing at the end of the session is a beneficial source of energy for your body.

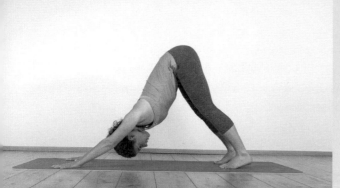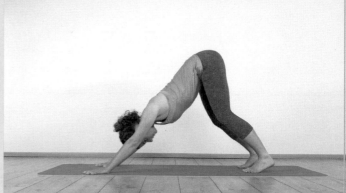

1 and 2. Dancing dog (see page 107)

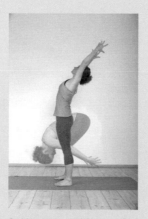

3. Mountain and forward fold
(see page 122)

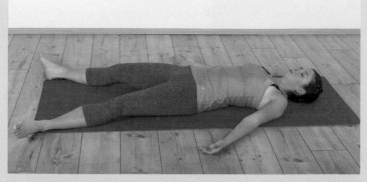

Final relaxation (see page 134)

Fascia yoga for runners

This sequence for runners or walkers focuses on swinging, bouncing elements to bring elasticity back to the fascia after it has been subjected to monotonous stress. You start the sequence by rolling the legs, then warm up with the fascia salutation. The "Strong and stable" flow is fully focused on strengthening and stabilising your core. After the swinging elements, there are a few exercises to bring length to your fascial network.

Arriving: Take two to three minutes to arrive on your mat. Close your eyes and concentrate on your breathing and on maintaining an upright sitting position.

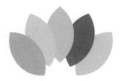

Breathing

Begin the session with a breathing exercise. You will notice that these first few minutes during which you focus all your awareness on yourself bring calm. Your breathing becomes more conscious, the breaths a little deeper, and your fascia yoga session more intense and effective.

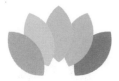

Releasing tension

Self-massage with a fascia roller and fascia balls is a wonderful start to a fascia yoga practice. This rolling stimulates the blood flow to the muscle and fascial tissues and gently releases tensions and even painful stuck areas. I have already presented the basic principles in chapter 4. Rolling selected parts of the body is the perfect way to prepare the body for various yoga exercises, so that they become even more intense and beneficial.

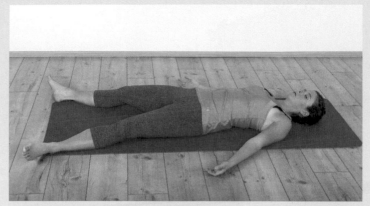

Full yoga breathing (see page 131)

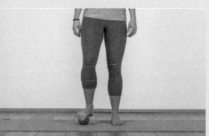

1. Soles of the feet (see page 31)

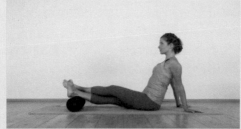

2. Achilles tendons (see page 33)

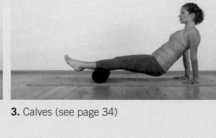

3. Calves (see page 34)

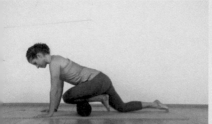

4. Shins (see page 35)

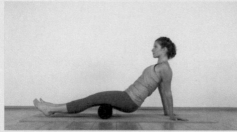

5. Hamstrings (see page 37)

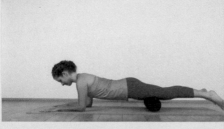

6. Thighs (see page 36)

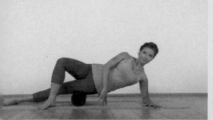

7. Outer thighs (see page 38)

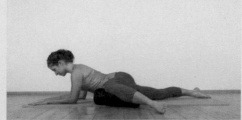

8. Inner thighs (see page 39)

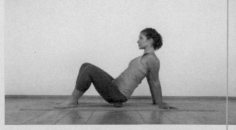

9. Buttocks with roller and/or ball (see page 40)

Special sequences for runners

Classic fascia salutation

The fascia salutation follows the major principles of the yoga poses in the sun salutation, but includes additional elements of fascia yoga. You stretch, bounce and jump in three dimensions. We use the exercises from the sections "Lengthen and extend", "Strong and stable" and "Swing, bounce and jump". You have already been introduced to all the exercises in previous chapters.

Classic fascia salutation plus

Expand the classic fascia salutation with powerful dynamic elements that you have already seen in the sections "Lengthen and extend" and "Swing, bounce and jump". Moving from downward-facing dog, move one leg forward into high lunge. From here, you can include various warrior and triangle variations, bringing even more elastic elements (swinging warrior and springing dog) into the fascia salutation.

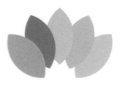

Strong and stable

The core is key to our posture and movements. The deep fascial chain acts as our internal stabiliser. Without it, our posture would be unstable and our movements weak. I have put together a short but very intense flow for you that reaches the core and requires strength in the arms and shoulders.

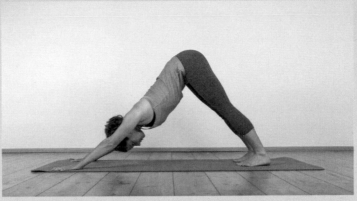

Classic fascia salutation (see pages 138–39); repeat four times

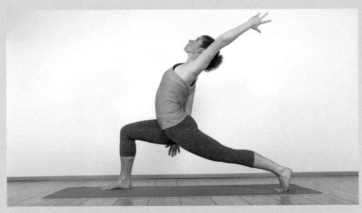

Classic fascia salutation plus (see pages 140–42); repeat four times

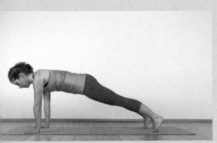

1. Exhale to high plank (see page 96)

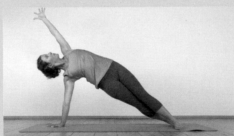

2. Inhale to side plank on right, hold for two breaths (see page 98)

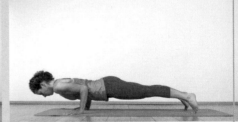

3. Exhale to low plank (see page 97)

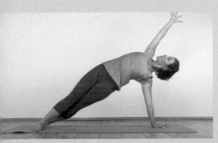

4. Inhale to side plank on left, hold for two breaths (see page 98)

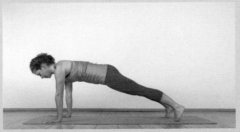

5. Exhale to high plank (see page 96)

Special sequences for runners

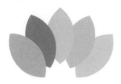

Additional follow-up exercises

Add to this flow with poses that again strengthen the core in a targeted way (boat, half boat and windscreen wipers). Hold them for five to ten breaths. Practice makes perfect. You will notice that you can gradually increase the number of breaths, or repeat the exercises two or three times.

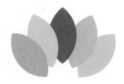

Swing, bounce and jump

Now it's time to be dynamic. The exercises selected bring elasticity to your fascial network. Energetic swinging, loose pulsing and lively springing movements promote collagen synthesis in the fascial tissue and ensure firm but flexible fascia.

The exercises selected focus on the fascia in the legs and back, which become inflexible from running.

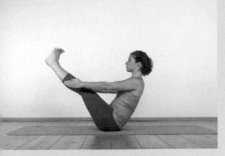

1. Boat (see page 99)

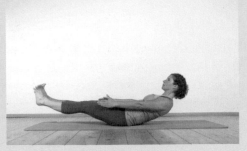

2. Half boat (see page 99)

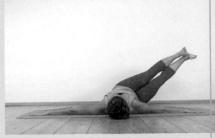

3. Windscreen wipers (see page 100)

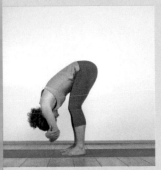

1. Pulsing forward fold
(see page 109)

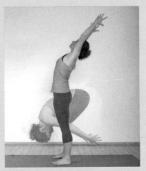

2. Mountain and forward fold
(see page 122)

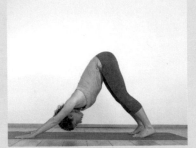

3. Dancing dog with pulsing heels
(see page 107)

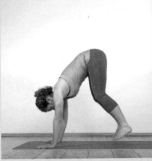

4. Springing dog into forward
fold (see page 117)

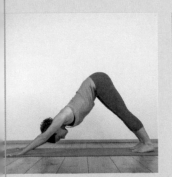

5. Downward-facing dog and
forward fold (see page 55)

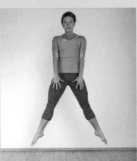

6. Frog jump (see page 119)

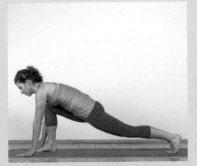

7. Jumping lunge (see page 120)

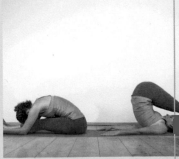

8. Rolling plow (see page 125)

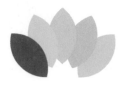

Lengthen and extend

Our fascia loves to be stretched out. With these carefully selected exercises, you can reach all the fascial chains that run through the body. Stay active in the poses, either by constantly changing the tensile load or by including small, gentle swinging movements. After these exercises, your body will feel much more supple and mobile.

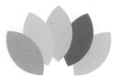

Relaxing stretches

After tensing, don't forget to relax at the end of your session. The relaxing stretches at the end of a session release and harmonise the structures you have been working. Take at least ten breaths, or even longer, to stay in the poses.

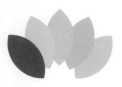

Final relaxation

Take five to ten minutes at the end of each session to relax in corpse pose, in order to allow your body, breathing and mind to come back to a calm state after the practice. Relaxing at the end of the session is a beneficial source of energy for your body.

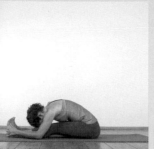
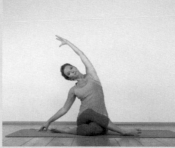
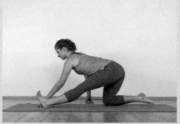
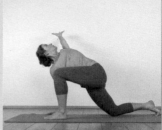

1. Pulsing seated forward fold (see page 53)

2. Shoelace with side bend (see page 73)

3. Half pyramid with exploring (see page 58)

4. Revolved side angle with opening (see page 81)

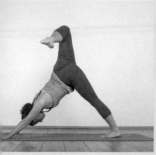
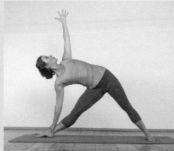
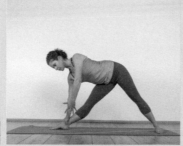
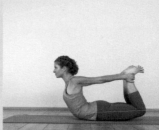

1. Three-legged dog with twist (see page 83)

2. Triangle (see page 76)

3. Circling triangle (see page 76)

4. Bow (see page 68)

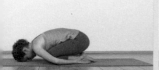
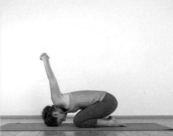
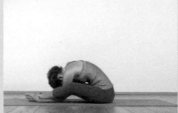
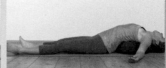

1. Child (see page 59)

2. Child with clasped hands (see page 91)

3. Tortoise (see page 102)

4. Fish using a meditation cushion (see page 70)

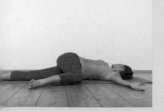
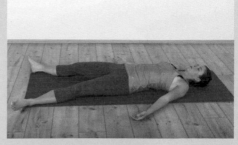

5. Knee down twist (see page 86)

Final relaxation (see page 134)

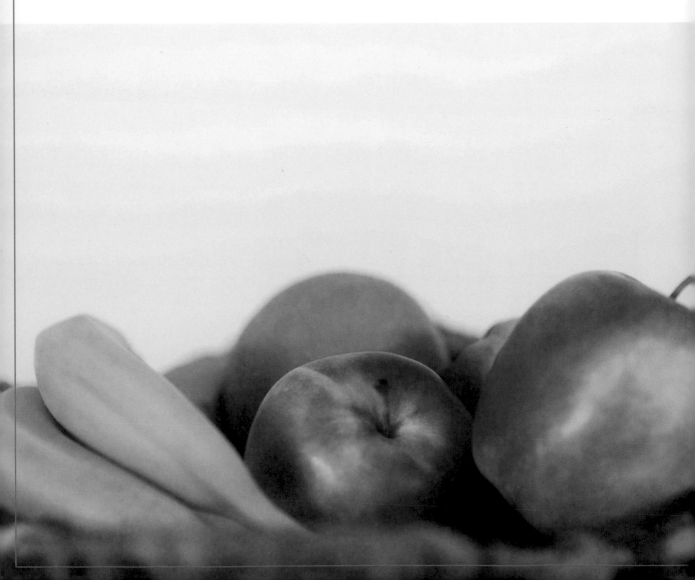

Chapter 10

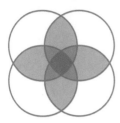

More things fascia loves

Last, but not least, I would like to give you a few more tips on caring for your fascia. So you can look after it off the yoga mat, too.

Move, move, move

Fascia loves nothing more than being moved – in as many different ways as possible. Build elements of fascia training into your daily routine: go up and down the stairs with ease and suppleness, bounce up and down on your heels as you clean your teeth, and start the day with a good fascial stretch before you get out of bed.

Farewell to stress!

When the equilibrium between tension and relaxation is permanently shifted towards tension, the body reacts to this situation of constant stress by releasing stress hormones. Fascia researchers have determined that an increased level of stress hormones, particularly cortisol, impairs the formation of collagen, an important part of the fascial tissue. Stress permanently reduces fascia mobility and also affects the many nerve endings found in fascia, causing them to send pain signals.

Drink lots

Connective tissues are more than 50% water (chapter 2, "Ground substance"). Water is a means of transport and communication, and therefore essential for the metabolism in fascia. Drink plenty of still water after training and, of course, throughout the whole day.

Keep an eye on your acid–base balance

Being too acidic is not good for the body. And this is particularly true for fascia because of its high water content. Fascia becomes harder and the blood and lymph flows are impaired. This can lead to painful inflammation. We can counteract this with an anti-inflammatory alkaline diet (see below), breathing exercises to remove carbon dioxide (chapter 8) and getting enough sleep.

Anti-inflammatory foods

Herbal cooking: Herbs and spices have been used as plant-based "medicine" for hundreds of years, and for good reason. Ginger, turmeric, saffron, chamomile and liquorice are particularly good for dealing with inflammation. Hot spices like red pepper, chilli and paprika, as well as cinnamon and nutmeg, are antioxidative wonderfoods from our kitchens.

Fruit and vegetables: Vegetables have lots of secondary plant compounds, which also have an antioxidative effect. All red fruits and vegetables (tomatoes, grapefruit, watermelon, etc.) contain lots of carotenoids. All brassica vegetables (broccoli, Brussels sprouts, cauliflower, etc.) and berries, cherries, pomegranates and red grapes also come highly recommended. The vitamin C content of citrus fruits and fruit peels has a positive effect on the body, reducing inflammation. And garlic and onions are anti-inflammatory too.

Good fats: Avoid saturated fatty acids, found above all in animal products. Polyunsaturated fatty acids, mainly found in olive oil, sunflower oil and linseed oil, are good.

Drinks: Tea and red wine contain catechins, plant-based free-radical inhibitors, which protect the body from cell damage.

Avoid toxins and drugs

Nicotine consumption has a clear negative impact on blood circulation and blood oxygen content. This makes things easier for free radicals, and the toxins and waste products ultimately settle in the connective tissues.

Index